The Vibrant Keto Air Fryer Cookbook

Tasty and Delicious
Snacks & Appetizers Recipes

Rudy Kent

Introduction

What's the difference between an air fryer and deep fryer? Air fryers bake food at a high temperature with a high-powered fan, while deep fryers cook food in a vat of oil that has been heated up to a specific temperature. Both cook food quickly, but an air fryer requires practically zero preheat time while a deep fryer can take upwards of 10 minutes. Air fryers also require little to no oil and deep fryers require a lot that absorb into the food. Food comes out crispy and juicy in both appliances, but don't taste the same, usually because deep fried foods are coated in batter that cook differently in an air fryer vs a deep fryer. Battered foods needs to be sprayed with oil before cooking in an air fryer to help them color and get crispy, while the hot oil soaks into the batter in a deep fryer. Flour-based batters and wet batters don't cook well in an air fryer, but they come out very well in a deep fryer.

The ketogenic diet is one such example. The diet calls for a very small number of carbs to be eaten. This means food such as rice, pasta, and other starchy vegetables like potatoes are off the menu. Even relaxed versions of the keto diet minimize carbs to a large extent and this compromises the goals of many dieters. They end up having to exert large amounts of willpower to follow the diet. This doesn't do them any favors since willpower is like a muscle. At some point, it tires and this is when the dieter goes right back to their old pattern of eating. I have personal experience with this. In terms of health benefits, the keto diet offers the most. The reduction of carbs forces your body to mobilize fat and this results in automatic fat loss and better health.

Feel free to mix and match the recipes you see in here and play around with them. Eating is supposed to be fun! Unfortunately, we've associated fun eating with unhealthy food. This doesn't have to be the case. The air fryer, combined with the Mediterranean diet, will make your mealtimes fun-filled again and full of taste. There's no grease and messy cleanups to deal with anymore. Are you excited yet?

You should be! You're about to embark on a journey full of air fried goodness

Table of Contents

Three Meat Cheesy Omelet

Cooking Time:

20 minutes

Serve :2

Ingredients:

1beef sausage, chopped
4 slices prosciutto, chopped
1oz salami, chopped
1 cup mozzarella cheese, grated
1eggs
1 green onion, chopped
1 tbsp ketchup
1 tsp fresh parsley, chopped

Directions:

1.Preheat air fryer to 350 F. Whisk the eggs with ketchup in a bowl. Stir in green onion, mozzarella, salami, and prosciutto.

2.AirFry the sausage in a greased baking tray in the fryer for 2 minutes. Slide-out and pour the egg mixture on top.

3.Cook for another 8 minutes until golden. Serve sliced with parsley

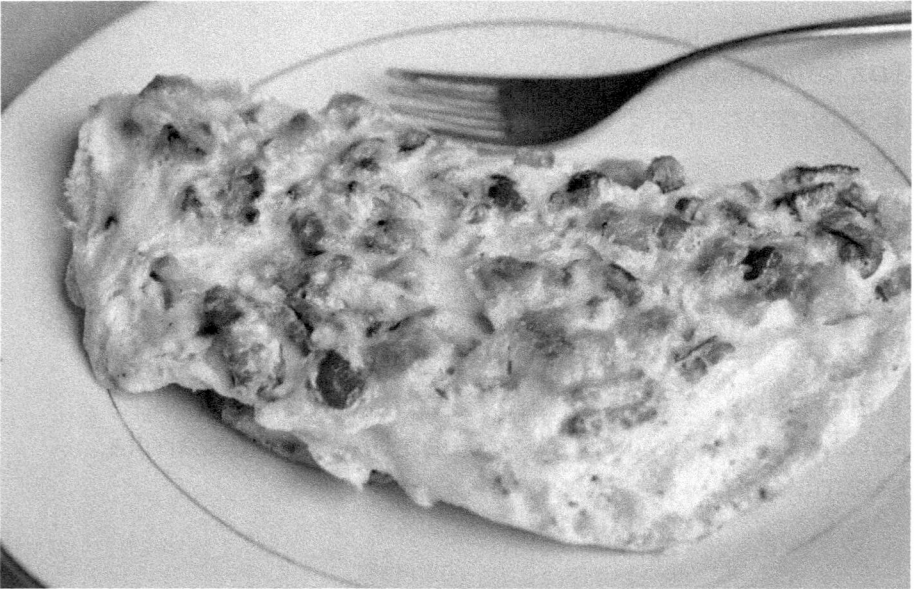

Orange Creamy Cupcakes

Cooking Time:

20 minutes

Serve:4

Ingredients

Lemon Frosting:
1 cup plain yogurt
2 tbsp sugar
1 orange, juiced
1 tbsp orange zest
7 oz cream cheese

Cake:

2 lemons, seeded and quartered

½ cup flour + extra for basing

¼ tsp salt

2 tbsp sugar

1 tsp baking powder

1 tsp vanilla extract

2 eggs

½ cup butter, softened 2 tbsp milk

Directions:

1.In a bowl, add yogurt and cream cheese and mix until smooth.

2.Add in orange juice and zest and whisk well. Gradually add the sugar and stir until smooth. Make sure the frost is not runny. Set aside.

3.Place the lemon quarters in a food processor and process until pureed. Add in the flour, baking powder, softened butter, milk, eggs, vanilla extract, sugar, and salt. Process again until smooth.

4.Preheat air fryer to 360 F. Flour the bottom of 4 cupcake cases and spoon the batter into the cases, ¾ way up.

5.Place them in the air fryer and bake for 12 minutes or until the inserted toothpick comes out clean. Once ready, remove and let cool. Design the cupcakes with the frosting and serve.

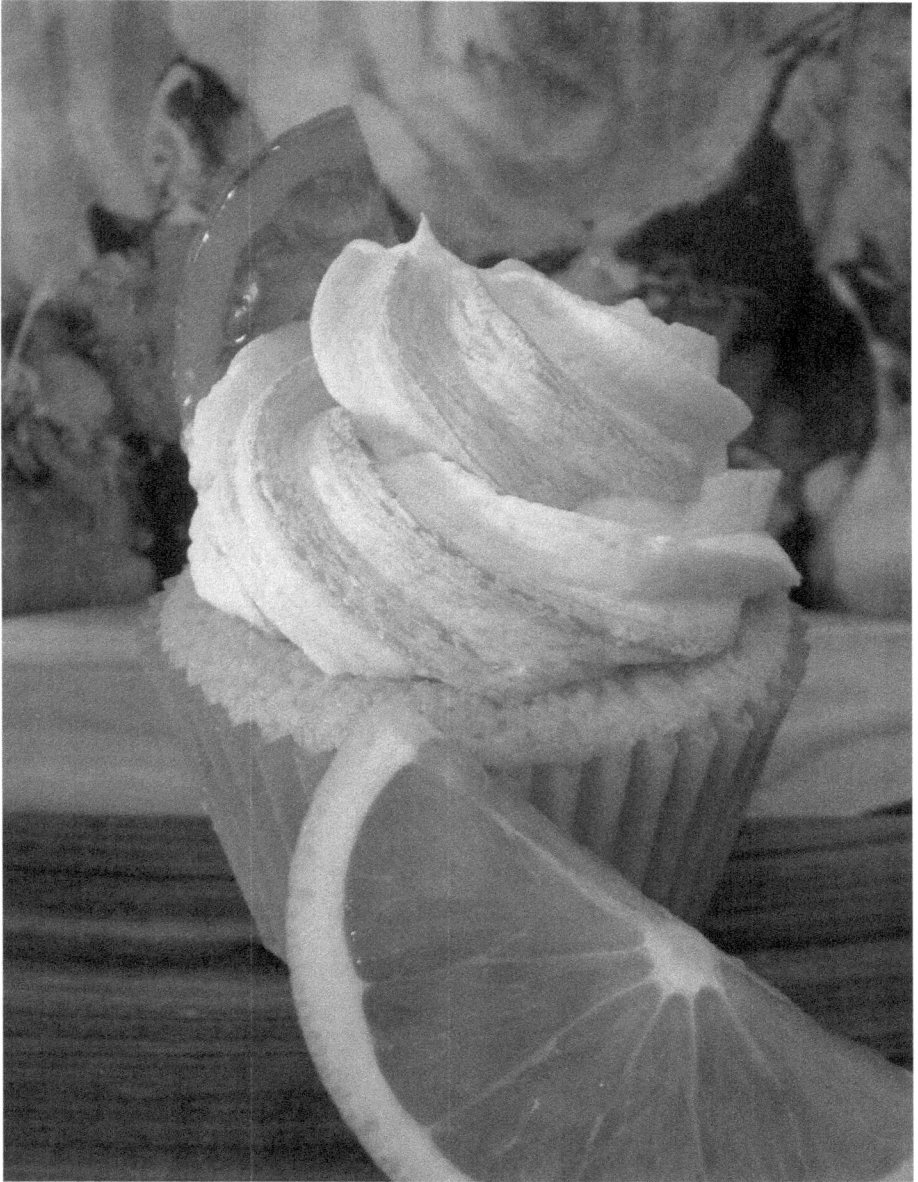

Avocado Tempura

Cooking Time:

10 minutes

Serve: 4

Ingredients:

½ cup breadcrumbs
½ tsp salt
1 avocado, pitted, peeled, and sliced
½ cup liquid from beans

Directions:

1.Preheat air fryer to 360 F. In a bowl, add the crumbs and salt and mix to combine.

2.Sprinkle the avocado with the beans' liquid and then coat in the crumbs.

3.Arrange the slices in one layer inside the fryer and Air Fry for 8-10 minutes, shaking once or twice. Serve warm

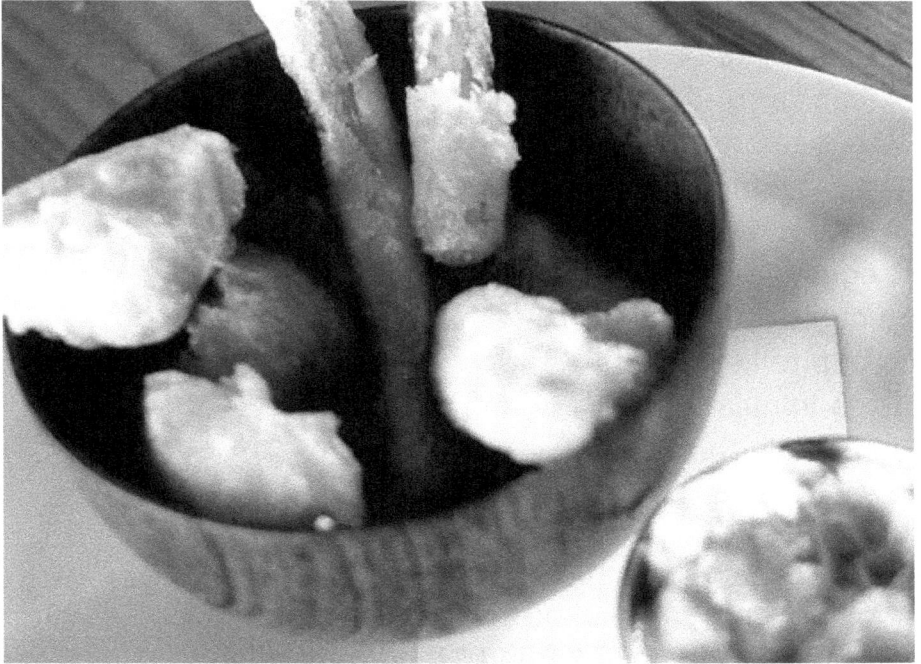

Blueberry Oat Bars

Cooking Time:

20 minutes

Serve: 12 bar

Ingredients:

1cups rolled oats
¼ cup ground almonds
¼ cup sugar
1 tsp baking powder
½ tsp ground cinnamon
2 eggs, lightly beaten
½ cup canola oil
½ cup milk
1 tsp vanilla extract
2 cups blueberries

Directions:

1.Spray a baking pan that fits in your air fryer with cooking spray. In a bowl, add oats, almonds, sugar, baking powder, and cinnamon and stir well.

2.In another bowl, whisk eggs, canola oil, milk, and vanilla. Stir the wet ingredients gently into the oat mixture.

3.Fold in the blueberries. Pour the mixture into the pan and place it in the fryer. Cook for 10 minutes at 350 F. Let it cool on a wire rack. Cut into 12 bars.

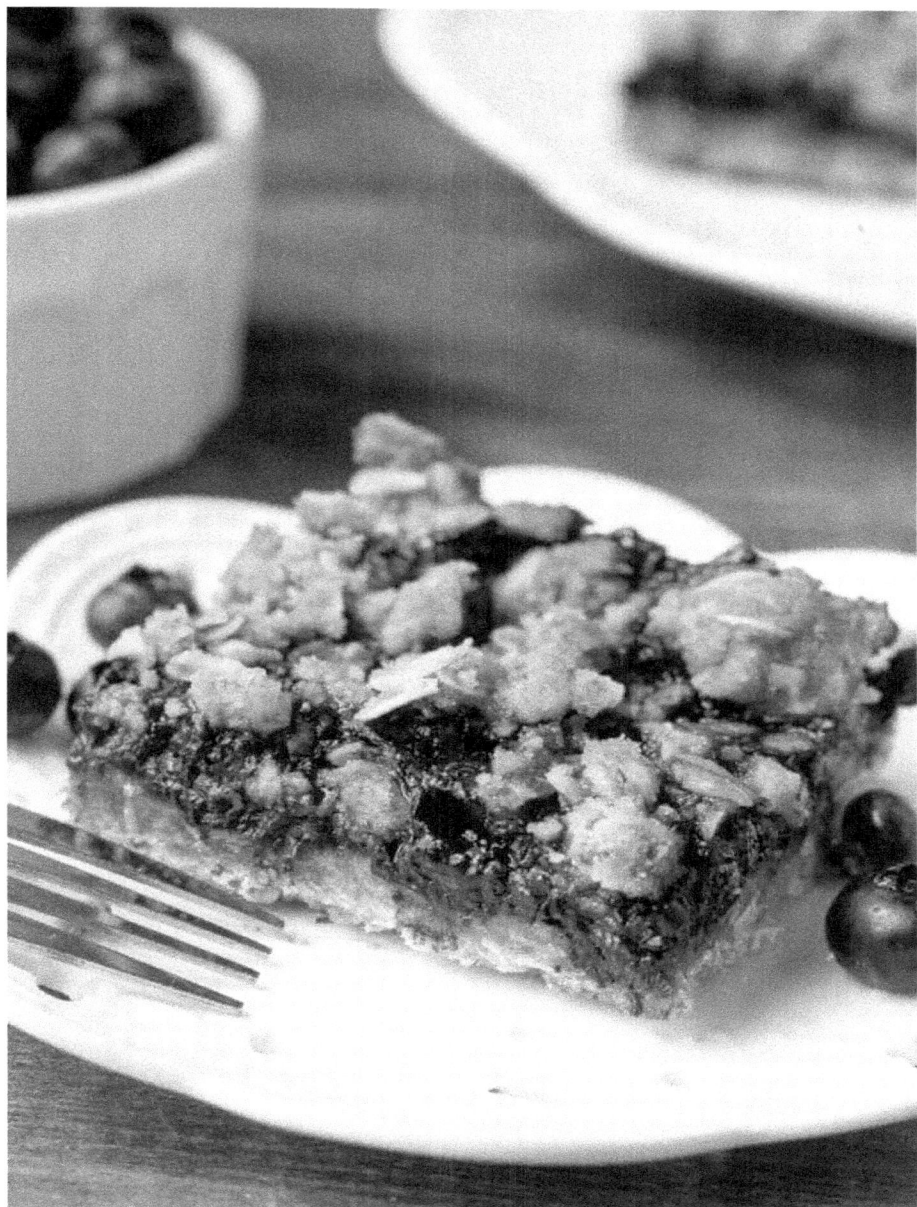

Crispy Croutons

Cooking Time:

20 minutes

Serve:4

Ingredients:

2 cups bread cubes
2 tbsp butter, melted
1 tsp dried parsley
Garlic salt and black pepper to taste

Directions:

1.Mix the cubed bread with butter, parsley, garlic salt, and black pepper until well coated.

2.Place in the fryer's basket and Air Fry for 6-8 minutes at 380 F, shaking once until golden brown. Use in soups.

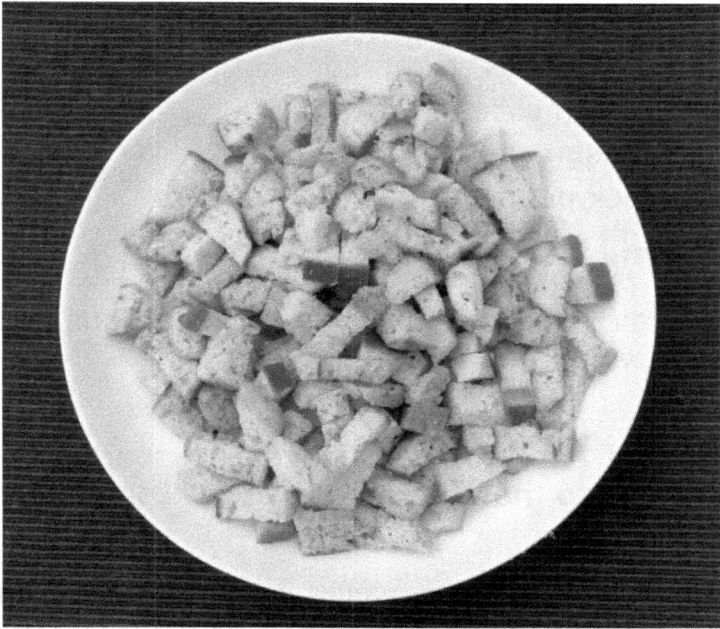

Roasted Asparagus with Serrano Ham

Cooking Time:

15 minutes

Serve:4

Ingredients:

12 spears asparagus, trimmed
12 Serrano ham slices
¼ cup Parmesan cheese, grated
Salt and black pepper to taste

Directions:

1.Preheat air fryer to 350 F. Season asparagus with salt and black pepper.

2.Wrap each ham slice around each asparagus spear from one end to the other end to cover completely.

3.Arrange them on the greased air fryer basket and Air Fry for 10 minutes, shaking once or twice throughout cooking.

4.When ready, scatter with Parmesan cheese and serve immediately.

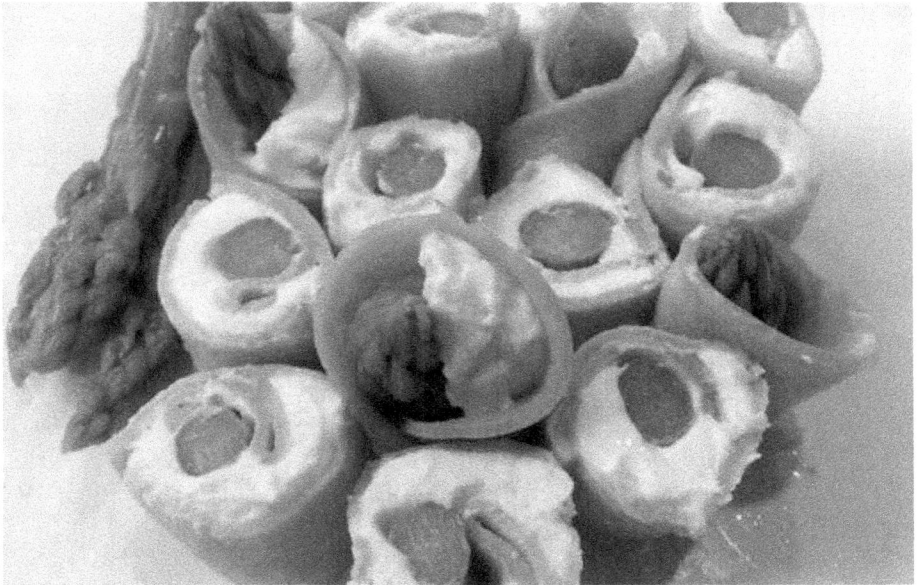

Very Berry Breakfast Puffs

Cooking Time:

20 minutes

Serve: 4

Ingredients:

1 puff pastry sheet
1 tbsp strawberries, mashed
1 tbsp raspberries, mashed
¼ tsp vanilla extract
1 cup cream cheese
1 tbsp honey

Directions:

1.Preheat air fryer to 375 F. Roll the puff pastry out on a lightly floured surface into a 1-inch thick rectangle.

2.Cut into 4 squares. Spread the cream cheese evenly on them.

3.In a bowl, combine the berries, honey, and vanilla. Spoon the mixture onto the pastry squares. Fold in the sides over the filling.

4.Pinch the ends to form a puff. Place the puffs on a lined with waxed paper baking dish.

5.Bake in the air fryer for 15 minutes until the pastry is puffed and golden all over. Let it cool for 10 mins before serving.

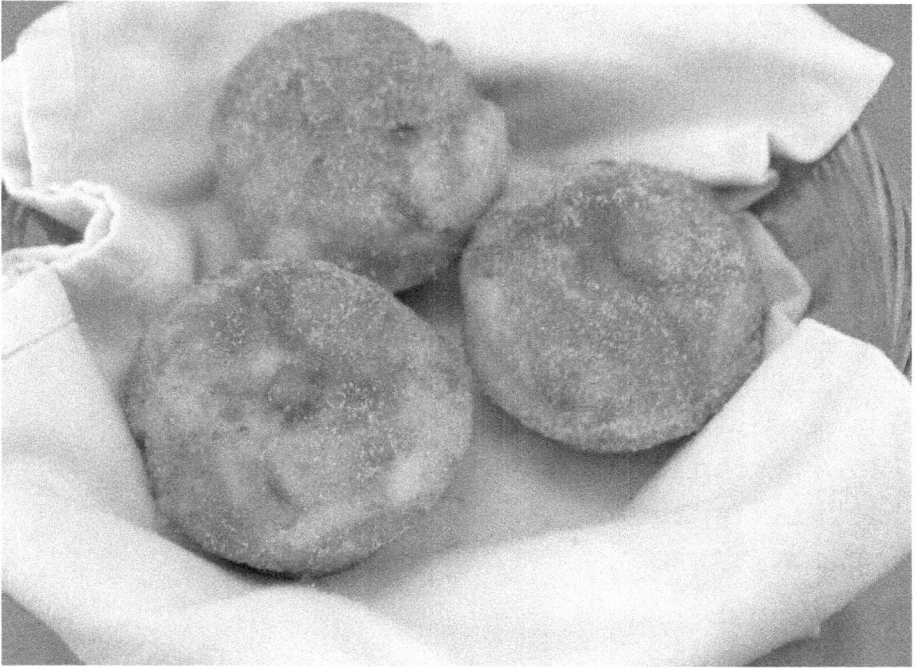

Mini Turkey and Corn Burritos

Cooking Time:

25 minutes

Serve:4

Ingredients:

1 tablespoon olive oil
½ pound ground turkey
2 tablespoons shallot, minced
1 garlic clove, smashed
1 red bell pepper, seeded and chopped
1 ancho chili pepper, seeded and minced
½ teaspoon ground cumin
Sea salt and freshly ground black pepper, to taste
⅓ cup salsa
6 ounces sweet corn kernels
12 8-inch tortilla shells
1 tablespoon butter, melted
½ cup sour cream, for serving

Directions:

1.Heat the olive oil in a sauté pan over medium-high heat. Cook the ground meat and shallots for 3 to 4 minutes.

2.Add the garlic and peppers and cook an additional 3 minutes or until fragrant. After that, add the spices, salsa, and corn.

3.Stir until everything is well combined. Place about 2 tablespoons of the meat mixture in the center of each tortilla.

4.Roll your tortillas to seal the edges and make the burritos. Brush each burrito with melted butter and place them in the lightly greased cooking basket.

5.Bake at 395 degrees F for 10 minutes, turning them over halfway through the cooking time. Garnish each burrito with a dollop of sour cream and serve.

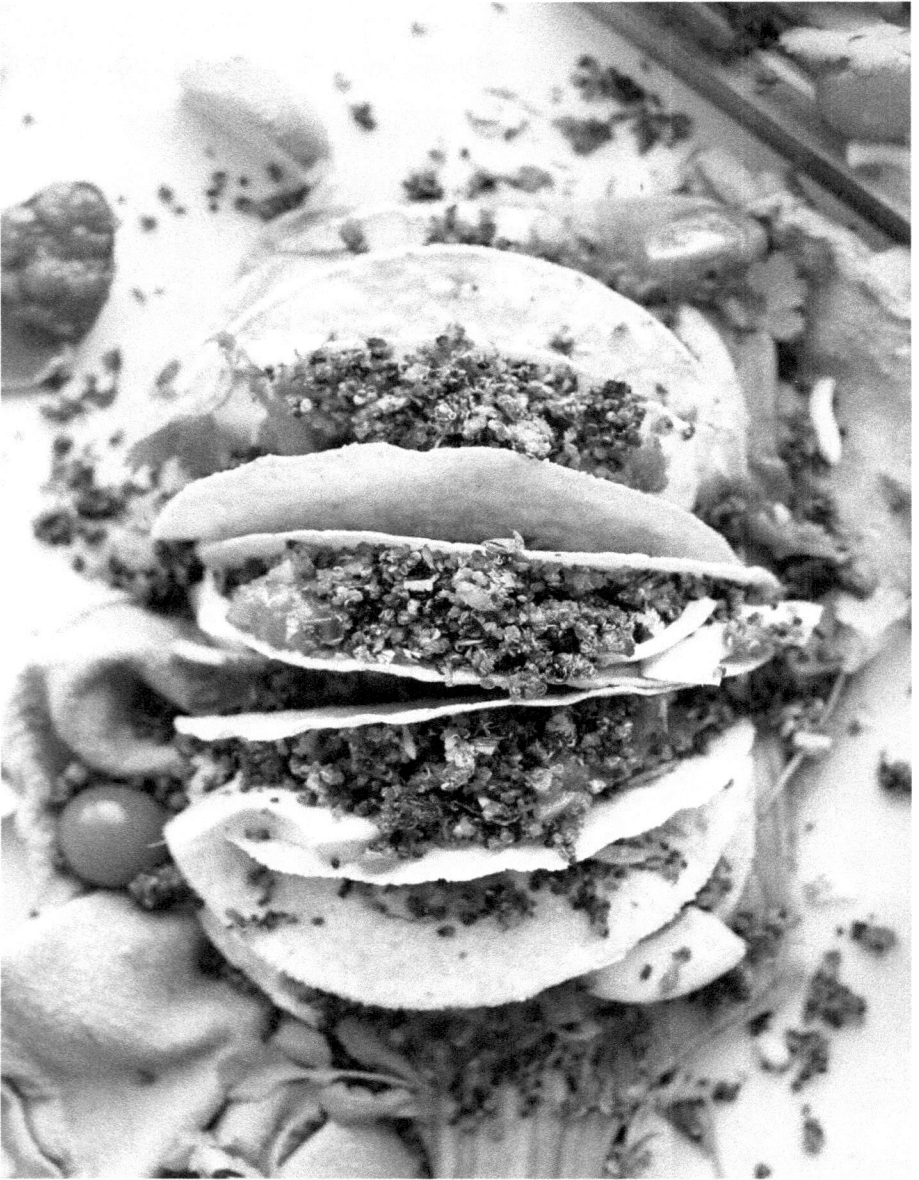

Cheddar Cheese Lumpia Rolls

Cooking Time:

20 minutes

Serve:4

Ingredients:

1 ounces mature cheddar cheese, cut into 15 sticks
15 pieces spring roll lumpia wrappers
2 tablespoons sesame oil

Directions:

1.Wrap the cheese sticks in the lumpia wrappers. Transfer to the Air Fryer basket. Brush with sesame oil.

2.Bake in the preheated Air Fryer at 395 degrees for 10 minutes or until the lumpia wrappers turn golden brown. Work in batches.

3.Shake the Air Fryer basket occasionally to ensure even cooking. Enjoy!

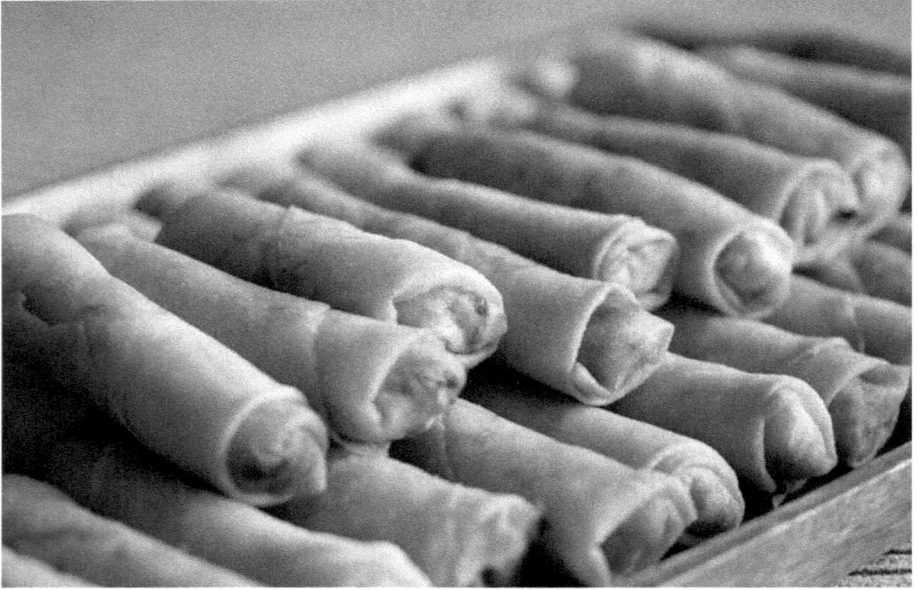

Spicy Korean Short Ribs

Cooking Time:

35 minutes

Serve:4

Ingredients:

1pound meaty short ribs
½ rice vinegar
½ cup soy sauce
1 tablespoon brown sugar
1 tablespoons Sriracha sauce
2 garlic cloves, minced
1 tablespoon daenjang soybean paste
1 teaspoon kochukaru chili pepper flakes
Sea salt and ground black pepper, to taste
1 tablespoon sesame oil
¼ cup green onions, roughly chopped

Directions:

1.Place the short ribs, vinegar, soy sauce, sugar, Sriracha, garlic, and spices in Ziploc bag; let it marinate overnight. Rub the sides and bottom of the Air Fryer basket with sesame oil.

2.Discard the marinade and transfer the ribs to the prepared cooking basket.

3.Cook the marinated ribs in the preheated Air Fryer at 365 degrees for 17 minutes.

4.Turn the ribs over, brush with the reserved marinade, and cook an additional 15 minutes. Garnish with green onions. Serve and enjoy!

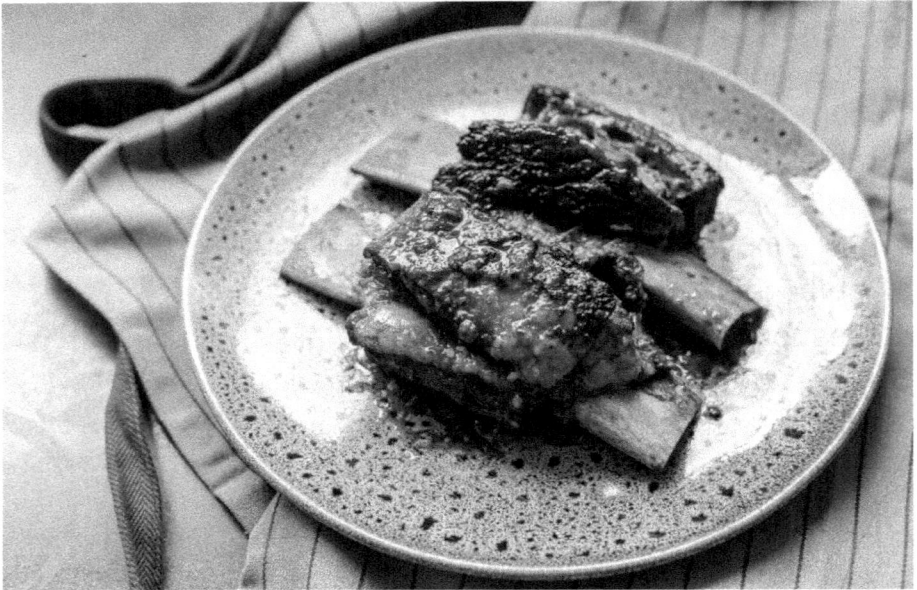

Crunchy Asparagus with Mediterranean Aioli

Cooking Time:

50 minutes

Serve: 4

Ingredients:

Crunchy Asparagus:
2 eggs
¾ cup breadcrumbs
2 tablespoons Parmesan cheese
Sea salt and ground white pepper, to taste
½ pound asparagus, cleaned and trimmed
Cooking spray

Mediterranean Aioli:

2   garlic cloves, minced

4 tablespoons olive oil mayonnaise

1 tablespoons lemon juice, freshly squeezed

Directions:

1.Start by preheating your Air Fryer to 400 degrees F. In a shallow bowl, thoroughly combine the eggs, breadcrumbs, Parmesan cheese, salt, and white pepper.

2.Dip the asparagus spears in the egg mixture; roll to coat well.

3.Cook in the preheated Air Fryer for 5 to 6 minutes; work in two batches. Place the garlic on a piece of aluminum foil and spritz with cooking spray.

4.Wrap the garlic in the foil. Cook in the preheated Air Fryer at 400 degrees for 12 minutes.

5.Check the garlic, open the top of the foil and continue to cook for 10 minutes more.

6.Let it cool for 10 to 15 minutes; remove the cloves by squeezing them out of the skins; mash the garlic and add the mayo and fresh lemon juice; whisk until everything is well combined.

7.Serve the asparagus with the chilled aioli on the side. Enjoy!

Cheesy Zucchini Sticks

Cooking Time:

20 minutes

Serve:4

Ingredients:

1 zucchini, slice into strips
2 tablespoons mayonnaise
¼ cup tortilla chips, crushed
¼ cup Romano cheese, shredded
Sea salt and black pepper, to your liking
1 tablespoon garlic powder
½ teaspoon red pepper flakes

Directions:

1.Coat the zucchini with mayonnaise. Mix the crushed tortilla chips, cheese and spices in a shallow dish.

2.Then, coat the zucchini sticks with the cheese/chips mixture. Cook in the preheated Air Fryer at 400 degrees F for 12 minutes, shaking the basket halfway through the cooking time.

3.Work in batches until the sticks are crispy and golden brown. Serve and enjoy!

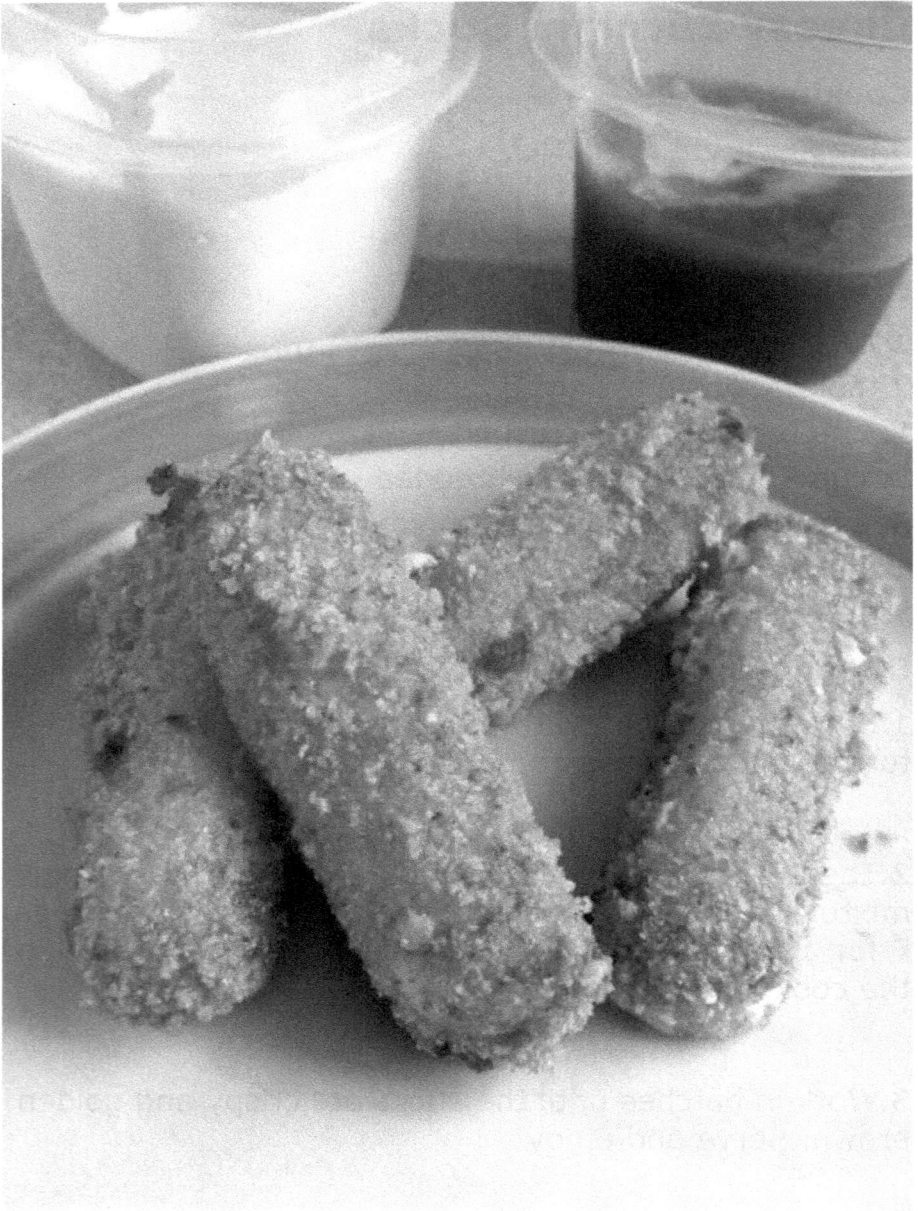

Parsnip Chips with Spicy Citrus Aioli

Cooking Time:

20 minutes

Serve:4

Ingredients:

1 pound parsnips, peel long strips
2 tablespoons sesame oil
Sea salt and ground black pepper, to taste
1 teaspoon red pepper flakes, crushed
½ teaspoon curry powder
½ teaspoon mustard seeds

Spicy Citrus Aioli:

¼ cup mayonnaise

1 tablespoon fresh lime juice

1 clove garlic, smashed

Salt and black pepper, to taste

Directions:

1.Start by preheating the Air Fryer to 380 degrees F. Toss the parsnip chips with the sesame oil, salt, black pepper, red pepper, curry powder, and mustard seeds.

2.Cook for 15 minutes, shaking the Air Fryer basket periodically.

3.Meanwhile, make the sauce by whisking the mayonnaise, lime juice, garlic, salt, and pepper. Place in the refrigerator until ready to use. Enjoy!

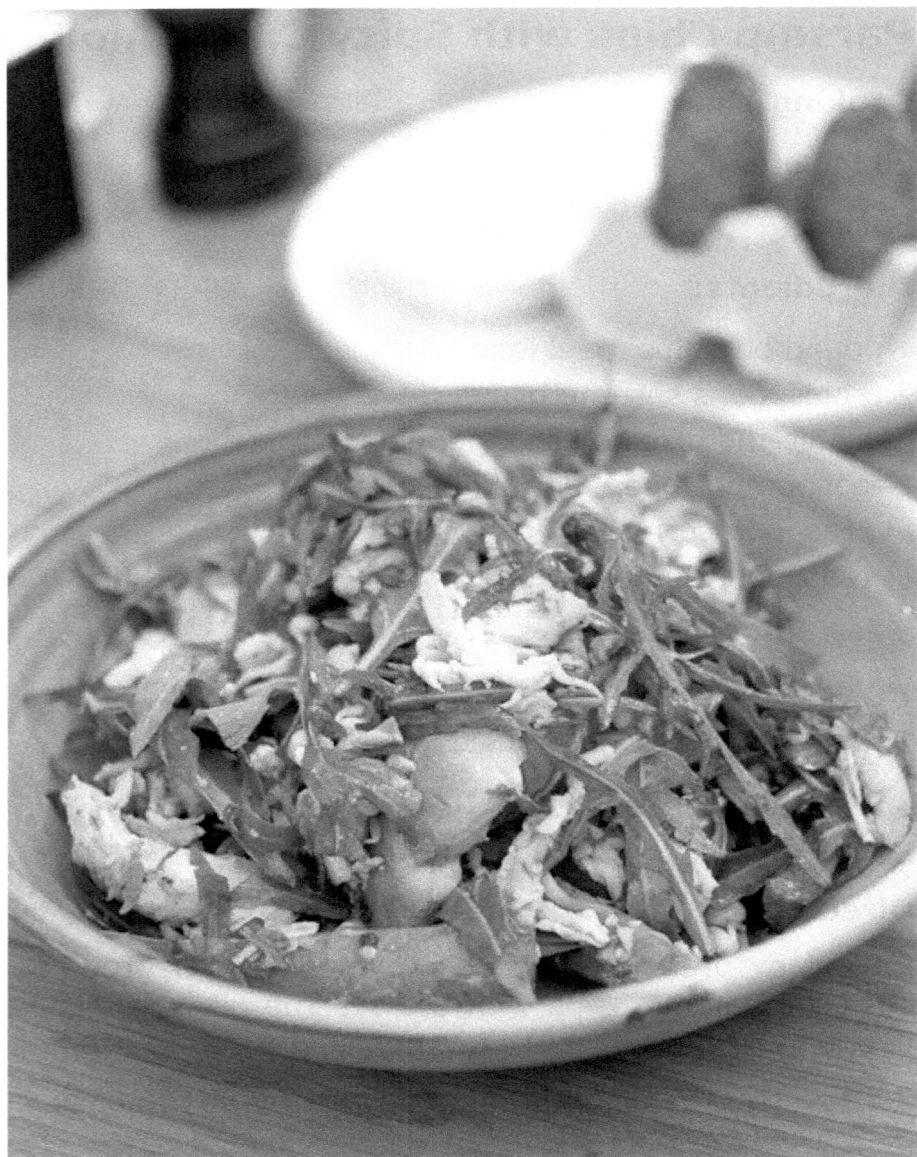

Bacon Chips with Chipotle Dipping Sauce

Cooking Time:

15 minutes

Serve:3

Ingredients:

 3 ounces bacon, cut into strips
Chipotle Dipping Sauce:
 4 tablespoons sour cream
½ teaspoon chipotle chili powder

Directions:

1.Place the bacon strips in the Air Fryer cooking basket.

2.Cook the bacon strips at 360 degrees F for 5 minutes; turn them over and cook for another 5 minutes.

3.Meanwhile, make the chipotle dipping sauce by whisking the sour cream and chipotle chili powder; reserve.

4.Serve the bacon chips with the chipotle dipping sauce and enjoy!

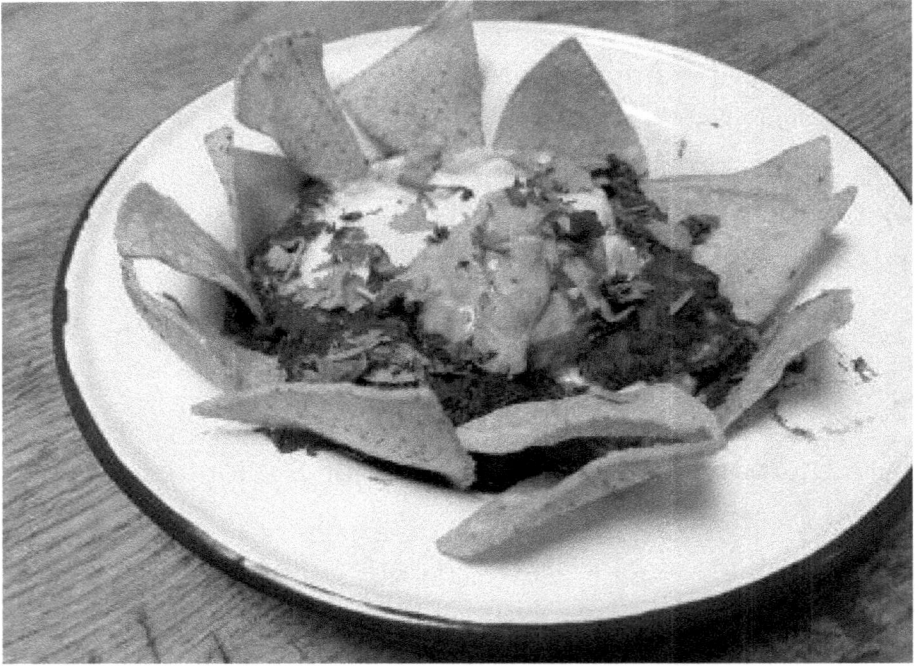

Fish Sticks with Honey Mustard Sauce

Cooking Time:

10 minutes

Serve:4

Ingredients:

10 ounces fish sticks
½ cup mayonnaise
2 teaspoons yellow mustard
2 teaspoons honey

Directions:

1.Add the fish sticks to the Air Fryer cooking basket; drizzle the fish sticks with a nonstick cooking spray.

2.Cook the fish sticks at 400 degrees F for 5 minutes; turn them over and cook for another 5 minutes.

3.Meanwhile, mix the mayonnaise, yellow mustard and honey until well combined. Serve the fish sticks with the honey mustard sauce for dipping. Enjoy!

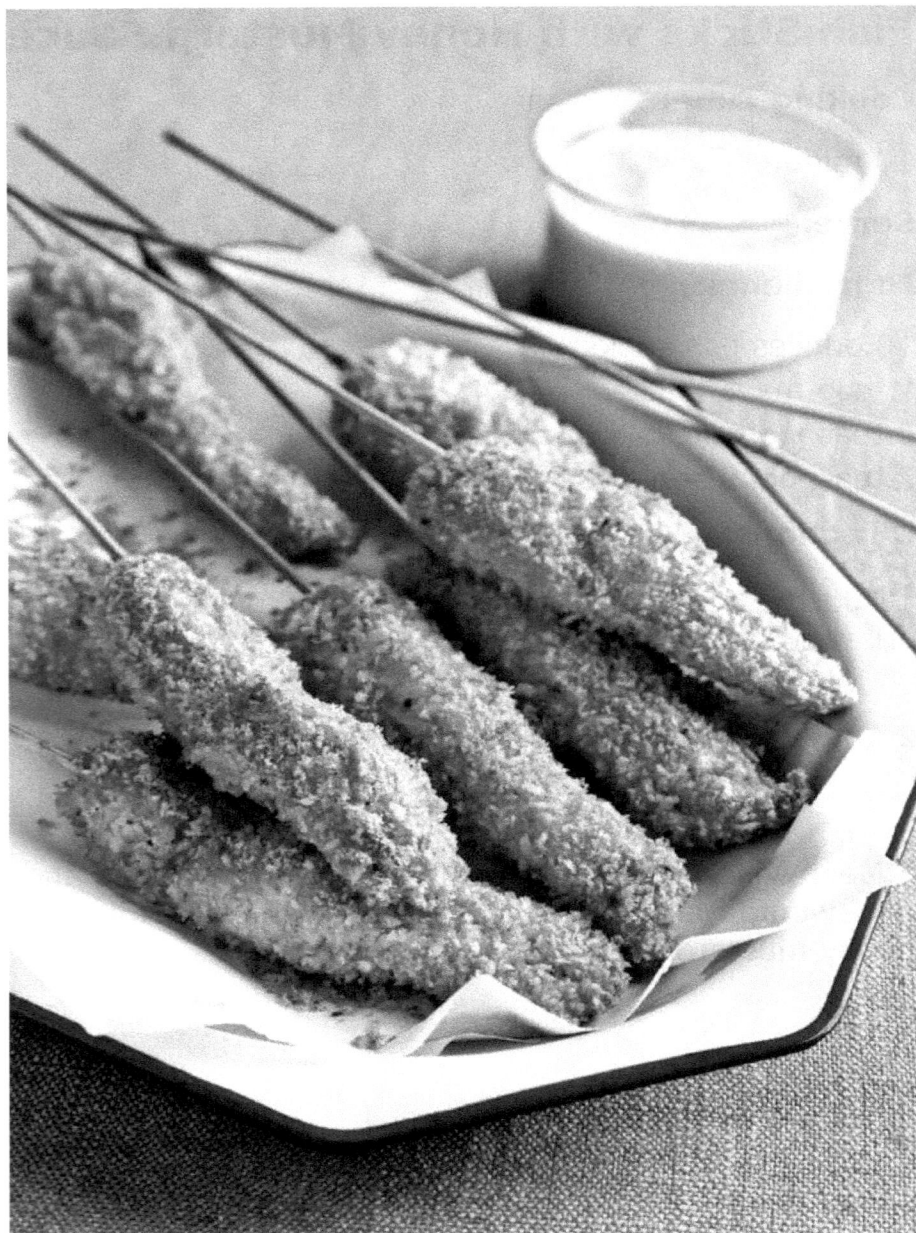

Mustard Brussels Sprout Chips

Cooking Time:

15 minutes

Serve:4

Ingredients:

½ pound Brussels sprouts, cut into small pieces
1 teaspoon deli mustard
1 teaspoon sesame oil
1 teaspoon champagne vinegar
¼ teaspoon paprika
¼ teaspoon cayenne pepper
Coarse sea salt and ground black pepper, to taste

Directions:

1.Start by preheating your Air Fryer to 360 degrees F. Toss the Brussels sprouts with the other ingredients until well coated. Transfer the Brussels sprouts to the

2.Air Fryer cooking basket. Cook the Brussels sprout chips in the preheated Air Fryer for about 20 minutes, shaking the basket every 6 to 7 minutes.

3.Serve with your favorite sauce for dipping. Enjoy!

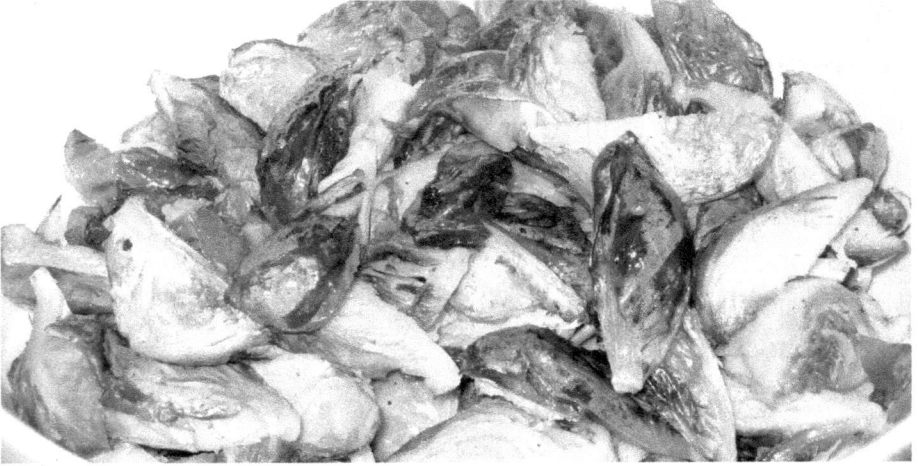

Avocado Fries with Chipotle Sauce

Cooking Time:

About 20 minutes

Servings: 3

Ingredients:

2tablespoons fresh lime juice

1 avocado, pitted, peeled, and sliced

Pink Himalayan salt and ground white pepper, to taste

¼ cup flour

1 egg

½ cup breadcrumbs

1 chipotle chili in adobo sauce

¼ cup light mayonnaise

¼ cup plain Greek yogurt

Directions:

1.Drizzle lime juice all over the avocado slices and set aside.

2.Then, set up your breading station. Mix the salt, pepper, and all-purpose flour in a shallow dish. In a separate dish, whisk the egg.

3.Finally, place your breadcrumbs in a third dish. Start by dredging the avocado slices in the flour mixture; then, dip them into the egg.

4.Press the avocado slices into the breadcrumbs, coating evenly.

5.Cook in the preheating Air Fryer at 380 degrees F for 11 minutes, shaking the cooking basket halfway through the cooking time.

6.Meanwhile, blend the chipotle chili, mayo, and Greek yogurt in your food processor until the sauce is creamy and uniform. Serve the warm avocado slices with the sauce on the side. Enjoy!

Spinach Chips with Chili Yogurt Dip

Cooking Time:

20 minutes

Serve:3

Ingredients:

2cups fresh spinach leaves
1 tablespoon extra-virgin olive oil
1 teaspoon sea salt
½ teaspoon cayenne pepper
1 teaspoon garlic powder
Chili Yogurt Dip:
¼ cup yogurt
2 tablespoons mayonnaise
½ teaspoon chili powder

Directions:

1.Toss the spinach leaves with the olive oil and seasonings.

2.Bake in the preheated Air Fryer at 350 degrees F for 10 minutes, shaking the cooking basket occasionally.

3.Bake until the edges brown, working in batches. In the meantime, make the sauce by whisking all ingredients in a mixing dish. Serve immediately.

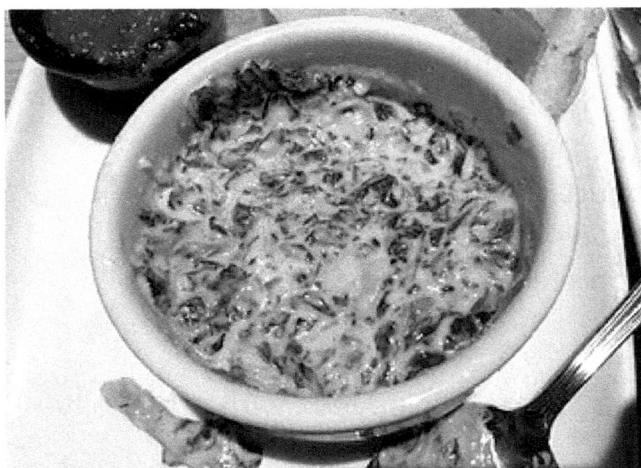

Crunchy Roasted Pepitas

Cooking Time:

20 minutes

Serve:3

Ingredients:

2 cups fresh pumpkin seeds with shells
1 tablespoon olive oil
1 teaspoon sea salt
1 teaspoon ground coriander
1 teaspoon cayenne pepper

Directions:

1.Toss the pumpkin seeds with the olive oil.

2.Spread in an even layer in the Air Fryer basket; roast the seeds at 350 degrees F for 15 minutes, shaking the basket every 5 minutes.

3.Immediately toss the seeds with the salt, coriander, salt, and cayenne pepper. Enjoy!

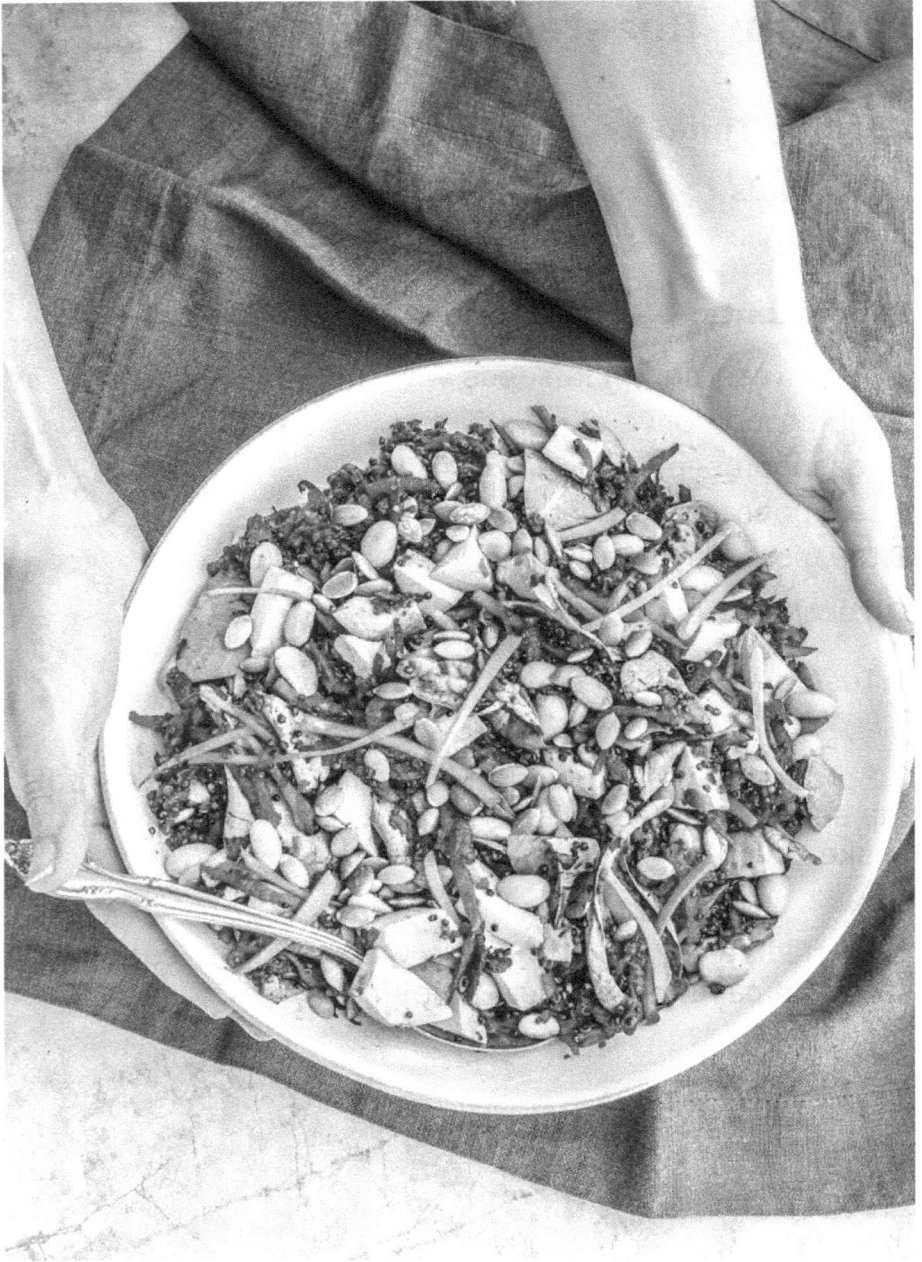

Loaded Tater Tot Bites

Cooking Time:

20 minutes

Serve:4

Ingredients:

24 tater tots, frozen
1 cup Swiss cheese, grated
6 tablespoons Canadian bacon, cooked and chopped
¼ cup Ranch dressing

Directions:

1.Spritz the silicone muffin cups with non-stick cooking spray.

2.Now, press the tater tots down into each cup. Divide the cheese, bacon, and Ranch dressing between tater tot cups.

3.Cook in the preheated Air Fryer at 395 degrees for 10 minutes. Serve in paper cake cups. Enjoy!

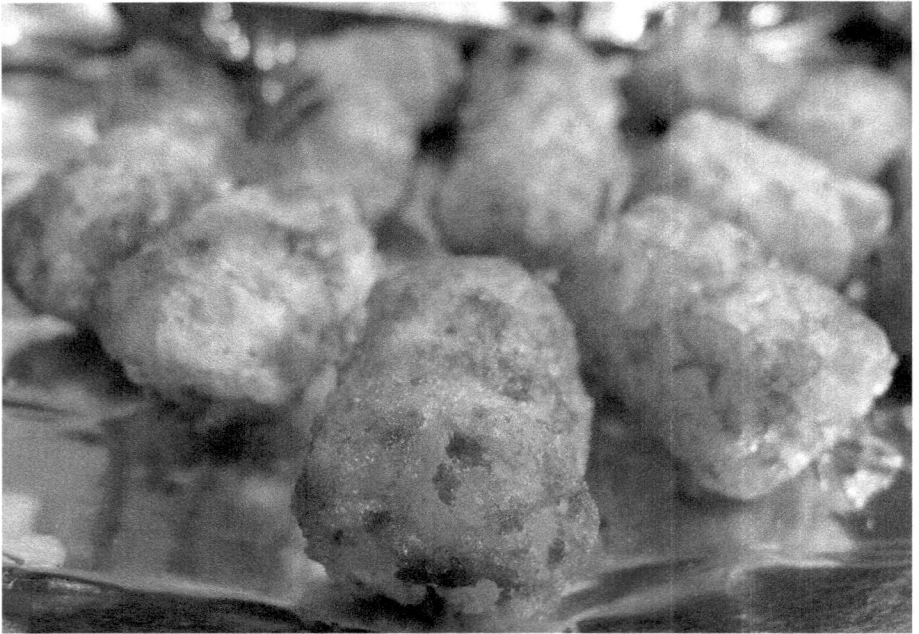

Classic Deviled Eggs

Cooking Time:

20 minutes

Serve: 3

Ingredients:

5 eggs
2 tablespoons mayonnaise
2 tablespoons sweet pickle relish
Sea salt, to taste
½ teaspoon mixed pepper corns, crushed

Directions:

1.Place the wire rack in the Air Fryer basket; lower the eggs onto the wire rack. Cook at 270 degrees F for 15 minutes.

2.Transfer them to an ice-cold water bath to stop the cooking.

3.Peel the eggs under cold running water; slice them into halves.

4.Mash the egg yolks with the mayo, sweet pickle relish, and salt; spoon yolk mixture into egg whites. Arrange on a nice serving platter and garnish with the mixed peppercorns. Enjoy!

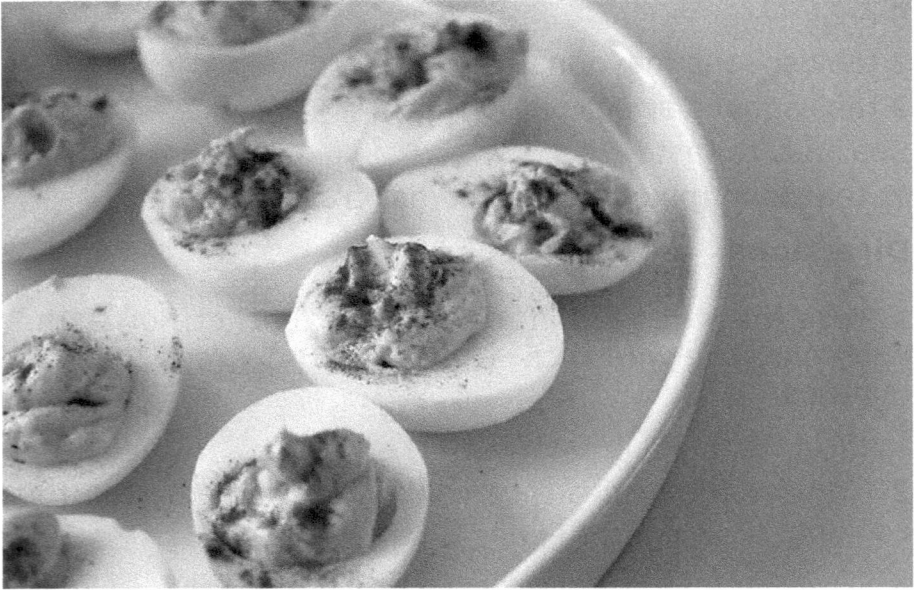

Green Bean Fries

Cooking Time:

20 minutes

Serve:6

Ingredients:

1egg, lightly beaten
1 lb green beans, ends trimmed
1/2 cup parmesan cheese, grated
1/2 tsp garlic powder
1 cup almond flour
1 tbsp mayonnaise
1/2 tsp garlic salt

Directions:

1.In a shallow bowl, whisk together egg and mayonnaise.

2.In a separate shallow bowl, mix together almond flour, parmesan cheese, garlic powder, and garlic salt. Place the cooking tray in the air fryer basket. Select Air Fry mode.

3.Set time to 10 minutes and temperature 390 F then press START. Roll green beans in egg then coat with almond flour mixture.

4.Spray breaded green beans with cooking spray. The air fryer display will prompt you to ADD FOOD once the temperature is reached then add breaded green beans in the air fryer basket.

5.Turn beans halfway through. Serve and enjoy.

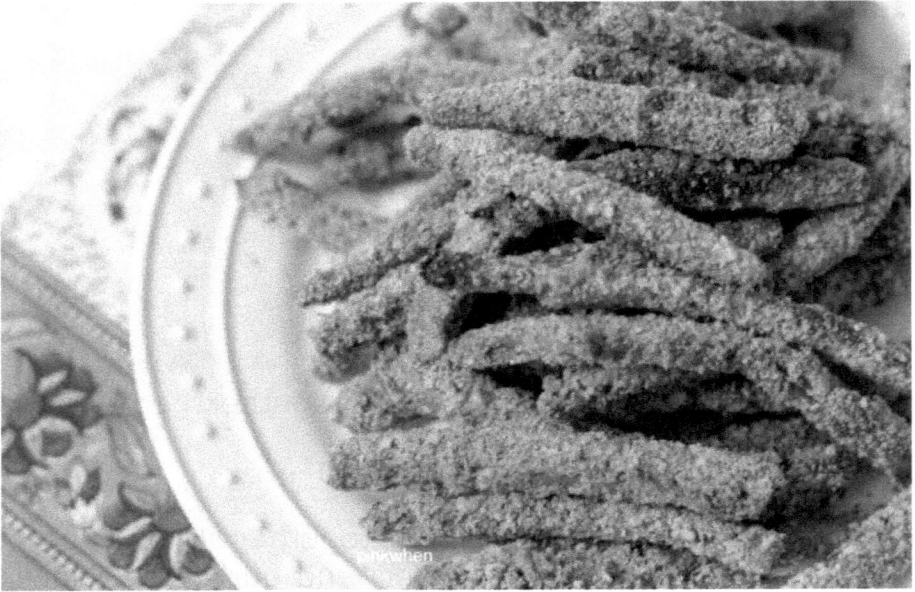

Quick & Delicious Biscuits

Cooking Time:

20 minutes

Serve:5

Ingredients:

1eggs
2 tbsp sour cream
2 tbsp butter, melted
1 cup cheddar cheese, shredded
1/2 tsp baking powder
1 cup almond flour
1/4 tsp pink Himalayan salt

Directions:

1.In a large bowl, mix together almond flour, cheddar cheese, baking powder, and salt until well combined.

2.Add sour cream, butter, and egg and mix until a sticky batter is formed. Place the cooking tray in the air fryer basket. Place piece of parchment paper into the air fryer basket.

3.Select Air Fry mode. Set time to 10 minutes and temperature 400 F then press START.

4.The air fryer display will prompt you to ADD FOOD once the temperature is reached then drop 1/4 cup sized of batter onto the parchment paper in the air fryer basket. Serve and enjoy.

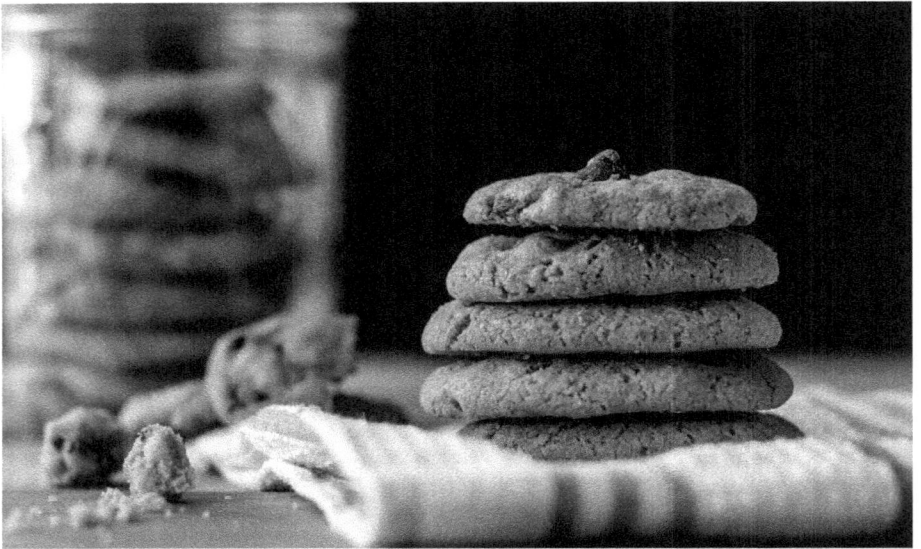

Tasty Zucchini Chips

Preparation Time:

10 minutes

Cooking Time:

12 minutes

Serve: 3

Ingredients:

1 egg, lightly beaten
1 large zucchini, cut into slices
3 tbsp roasted pecans, chopped
3 tbsp almond flour
1 tbsp Bagel seasoning

Directions:

1.In a small bowl, add egg and whisk lightly. In a shallow dish, mix together almond flour, chopped pecans, and bagel seasoning.

2.Dip zucchini slices into the egg then coat with almond flour mixture.

3.Place the cooking tray in the air fryer basket. Place piece of parchment paper into the air fryer basket. Select Air Fry mode.

4.Set time to 12 minutes and temperature 350 F then press START.

5.The air fryer display will prompt you to ADD FOOD once the temperature is reached then place zucchini slices onto the parchment paper in the air fryer basket.

6.Turn zucchini slices halfway through. Serve and enjoy.

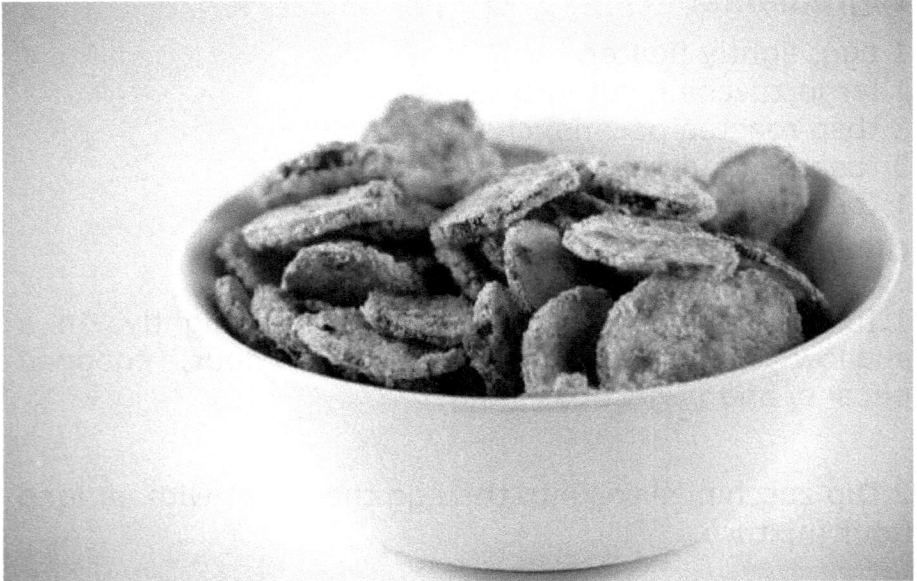

Perfect Cauliflower Tots

Preparation Time:

10 minutes

Cooking Time:

12 minutes

Serve: 4

Ingredients:

1 large cauliflower head, cut into florets

3 tbsp hot sauce

1/4 cup butter, melted

2 tbsp arrowroot

1 tbsp olive oil

Directions:

1.Toss cauliflower florets with olive oil and coat with arrowroot.

2.Place the cooking tray in the air fryer basket. Place piece of parchment paper into the air fryer basket.

3.Select Air Fry mode. Set time to 6 minutes and temperature 380 F then press START.

4.The air fryer display will prompt you to ADD FOOD once the temperature is reached then place cauliflower florets onto the parchment paper in the air fryer basket.

5.Meanwhile, in a mixing bowl, mix together hot sauce and melted butter. Once cauliflower florets are done then transfer them into the sauce and toss well.

6.Return cauliflower florets into the air fryer basket and air fry for 6 minutes more. Serve and enjoy.

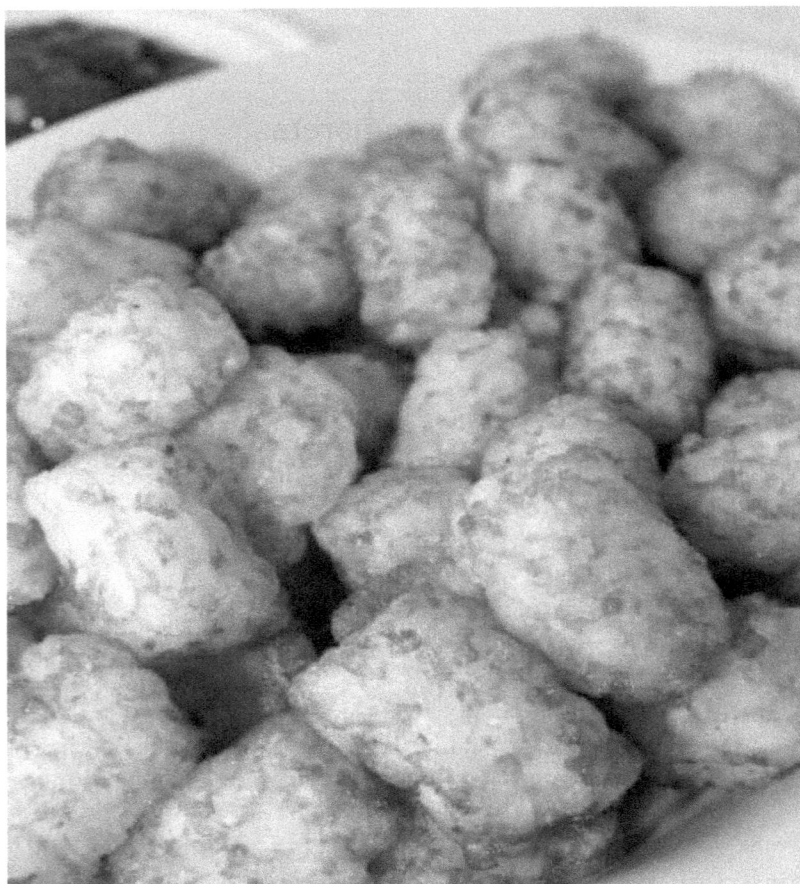

Crispy Air Fried Pickles

Preparation Time:

10 minutes

Cooking Time:

6 minutes

Serve: 4

Ingredients:

1 egg, lightly beaten
1/3 cup almond flour
16 dill pickle slices
1/4 cup parmesan cheese, grated
1/2 cup pork rinds, crushed

Directions:

1.In a small bowl, add egg and whisk well. In a separate bowl, add the almond flour.

2.In a shallow dish, mix together pork rinds and parmesan cheese.

3.Dredge pickle slices in almond flour mixture then egg and finally coat with crushed pork rind mixture.

4.Place the cooking tray in the air fryer basket. Place piece of parchment paper into the air fryer basket.

5.Select Air Fry mode. Set time to 6 minutes and temperature 370 F then press START.

6.The air fryer display will prompt you to ADD FOOD once the temperature is reached then place breaded pickle slices onto the parchment paper in the air fryer basket. Serve and enjoy.

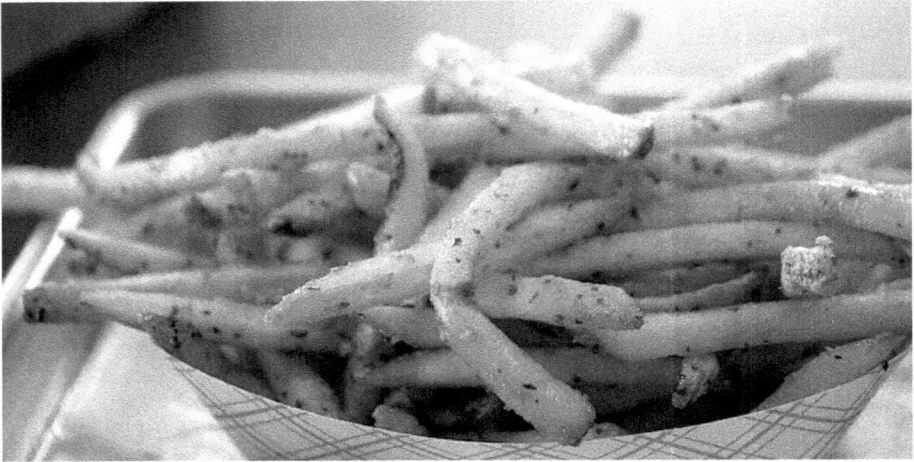

Asiago Asparagus Fries

Preparation Time:

10 minutes

Cooking Time:

10 minutes

Serve: 4

Ingredients:

1 lb asparagus spears, trim & cut in half
2 tbsp mayonnaise
2 oz asiago cheese, grated

Directions:

1.Add grated cheese in a shallow dish. Add asparagus and mayonnaise into the mixing bowl and mix well.

2.Coat asparagus spears with grated cheese. Place the cooking tray in the air fryer basket. Line air fryer basket with parchment paper.

3.Select Air Fry mode. Set time to 10 minutes and temperature 380 F then press START.

4.The air fryer display will prompt you to ADD FOOD once the temperature is reached then arrange asparagus spears onto the parchment paper in the air fryer basket. Serve and enjoy.

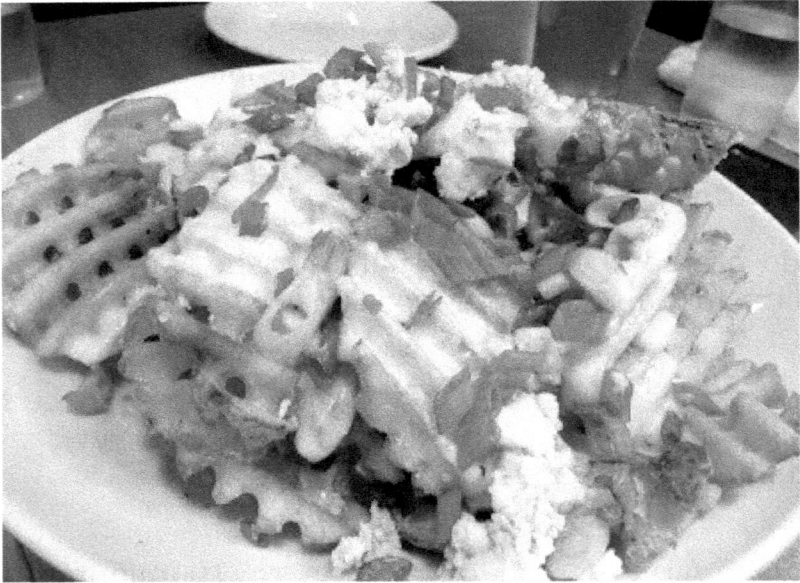

Crispy Air Fried Zucchini

Preparation Time:

10 minutes

Cooking Time:

15 minutes

Serve: 10

Ingredients:

1medium zucchini, sliced thinly lengthwise
1/4 cup mayonnaise
1 garlic clove, crushed
1/2 cup parmesan cheese, grated
1 cup pork rinds, crushed

Directions:

1.In a shallow dish, mix together crushed pork rinds and grated cheese.

2.In a mixing bowl, mix together zucchini slices, mayonnaise, and garlic.

3.Coat each zucchini slice with crushed pork rind mixture. Place the cooking tray in the air fryer basket. Line air fryer basket with parchment paper.

4.Select Air Fry mode. Set time to 15 minutes and temperature 350 F then press START.

5.The air fryer display will prompt you to ADD FOOD once the temperature is reached then place breaded zucchini slices onto the parchment paper in the air fryer basket. Serve and enjoy.

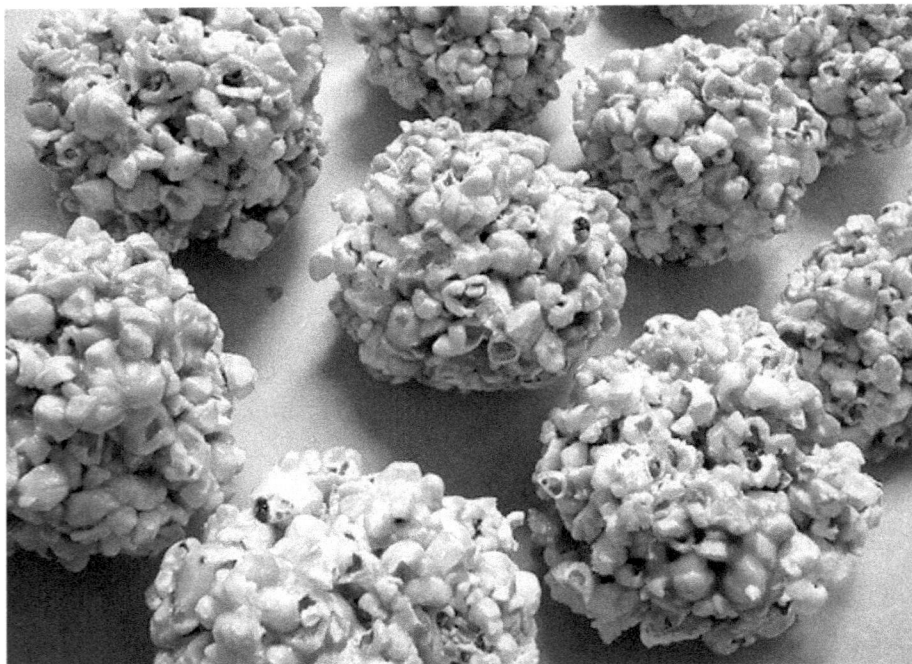

Cheese Balls

Preparation Time:

10 minutes

Cooking Time:

12 minutes

Serve: 8

Ingredients:

1eggs
1/2 tsp baking powder
1/2 cup almond flour
1/4 cup parmesan cheese, shredded
1/4 cup mozzarella cheese,shredded

1/2 cup cheddar cheese, shredded

Directions:

1.In a bowl, whisk eggs. Add remaining ingredients and mix until well combined.

2.Divide mixture into 8 equal portions. Roll each portion into a ball. Place the cooking tray in the air fryer basket.

3.Line air fryer basket with parchment paper. Select Bake mode. Set time to 12 minutes and temperature 400 F then press START.

4.The air fryer display will prompt you to ADD FOOD once the temperature is reached then place cheese balls onto the parchment paper in the air fryer basket. Serve and enjoy.

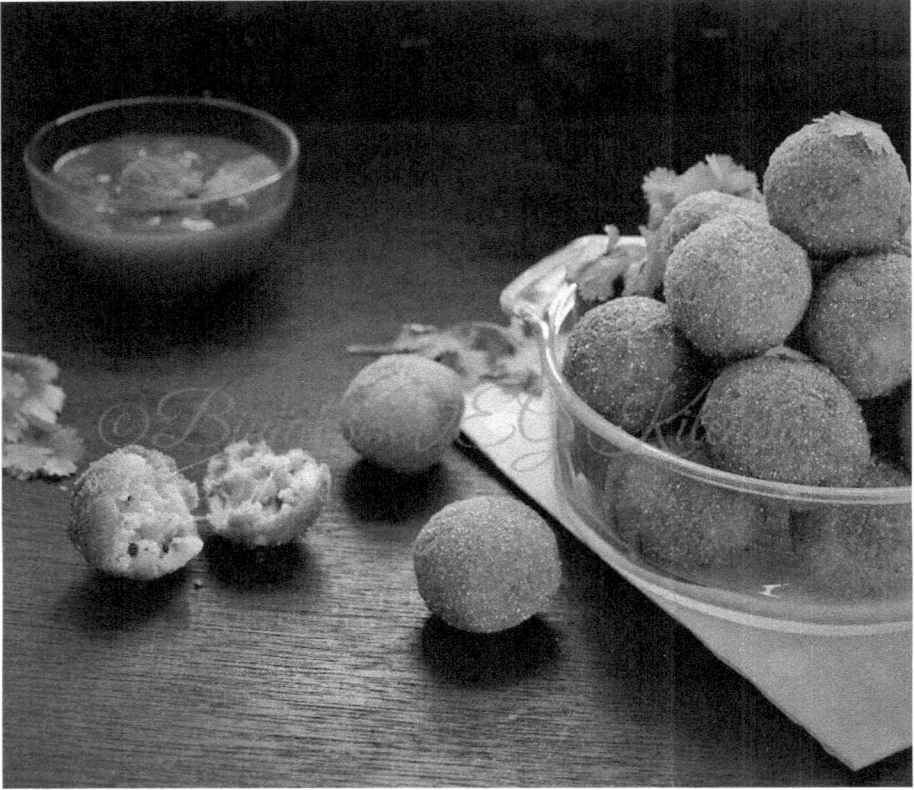

Chicken Meatballs

Preparation Time:

10 minutes

Cooking Time:

10 minutes

Serve: 6

Ingredients:

2eggs
3lbs ground chicken breast
1/2 cup almond flour
1/2 cup ricotta cheese
1/4 cup fresh parsley, chopped
1 tsp pepper
2 tsp salt

Directions:

1.Add all ingredients into the large bowl and mix until just combined. Make small balls from the meat mixture.

2.Place the cooking tray in the air fryer basket. Line air fryer basket with parchment paper. Select Air Fry mode.

3.Set time to 10 minutes and temperature 375 F then press START.

4.The air fryer display will prompt you to ADD FOOD once the temperature is reached then place meatballs onto the parchment paper in the air fryer basket. Serve and enjoy.

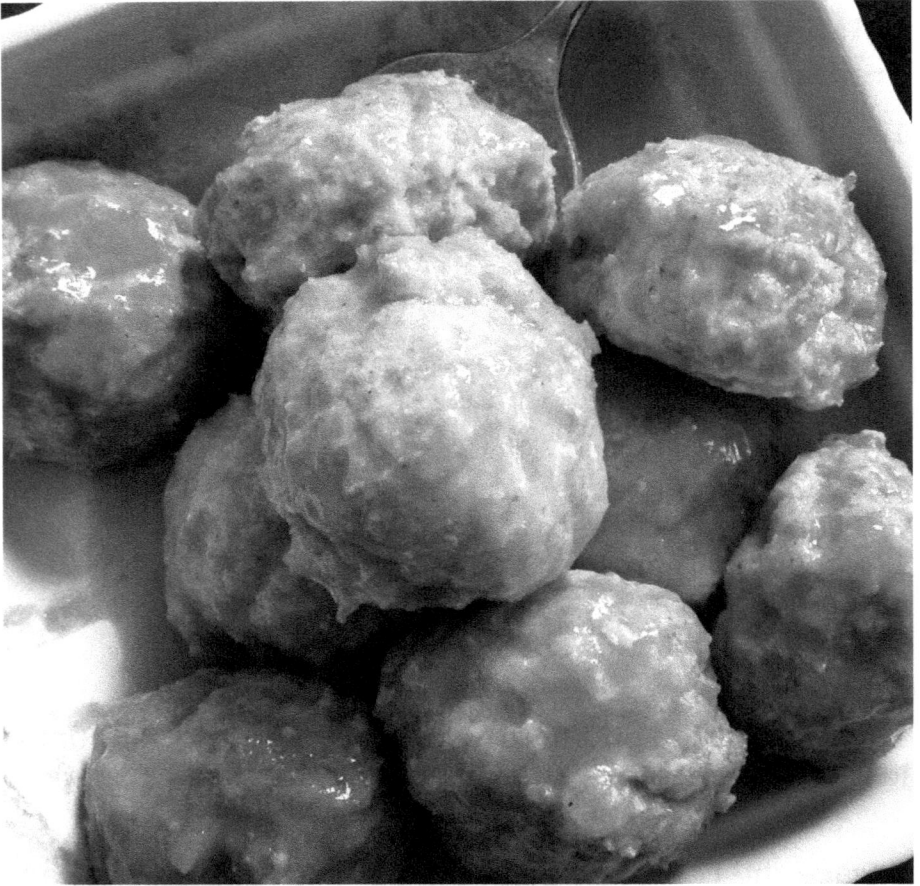

Garlic Dip

Preparation Time:

10 minutes

Cooking Time:

20 minutes

Serve: 12

Ingredients:

2garlic cloves, minced
5 oz Asiago cheese, shredded
1 cup sour cream
1 cup mozzarella cheese, shredded
8 oz cream cheese, softened

Directions:

1.Add all ingredients into the mixing bowl and mix until well combined. Pour mixture into the greased baking dish.

2.Select Bake mode. Set time to 20 minutes and temperature 350 F then press START.

3.The air fryer display will prompt you to ADD FOOD once the temperature is reached then place the baking dish in the air fryer basket. Serve and enjoy.

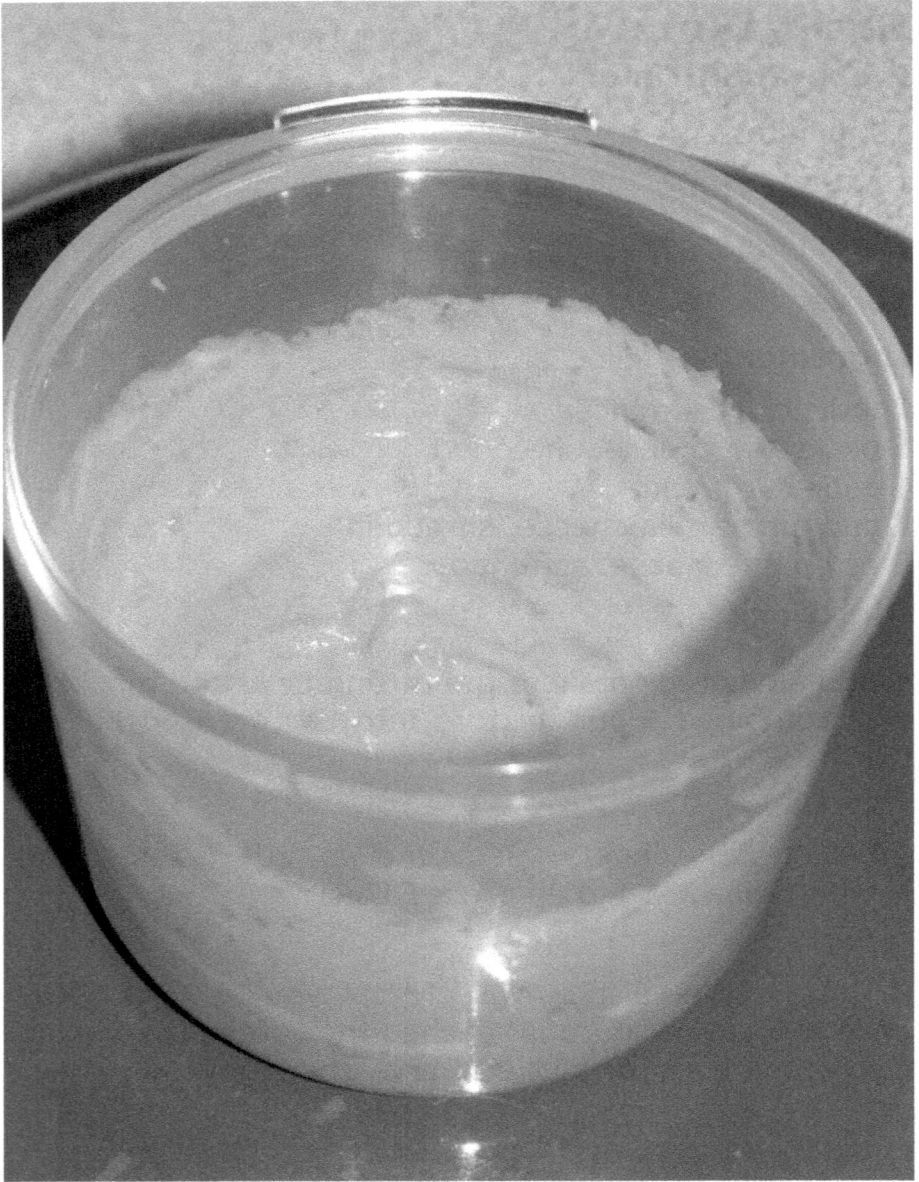

Crispy Tofu

Preparation Time:

10 minutes

Cooking Time:

15 minutes

Serve: 4

Ingredients:

15 oz extra-firm tofu, pressed and cut into cubes
1 tsp sesame oil
1 tbsp rice vinegar
2 tbsp soy sauce

Directions:

1.In a large bowl, mix together tofu, sesame oil, vinegar, and soy sauce. Let it sit for 15 minutes.

2.Place the cooking tray in the air fryer basket. Line air fryer basket with parchment paper. Select Bake mode.

3.Set time to 15 minutes and temperature 400 F then press START.

4.The air fryer display will prompt you to ADD FOOD once the temperature is reached then place tofu onto the parchment paper in the air fryer basket. Stir halfway through. Serve and enjoy.

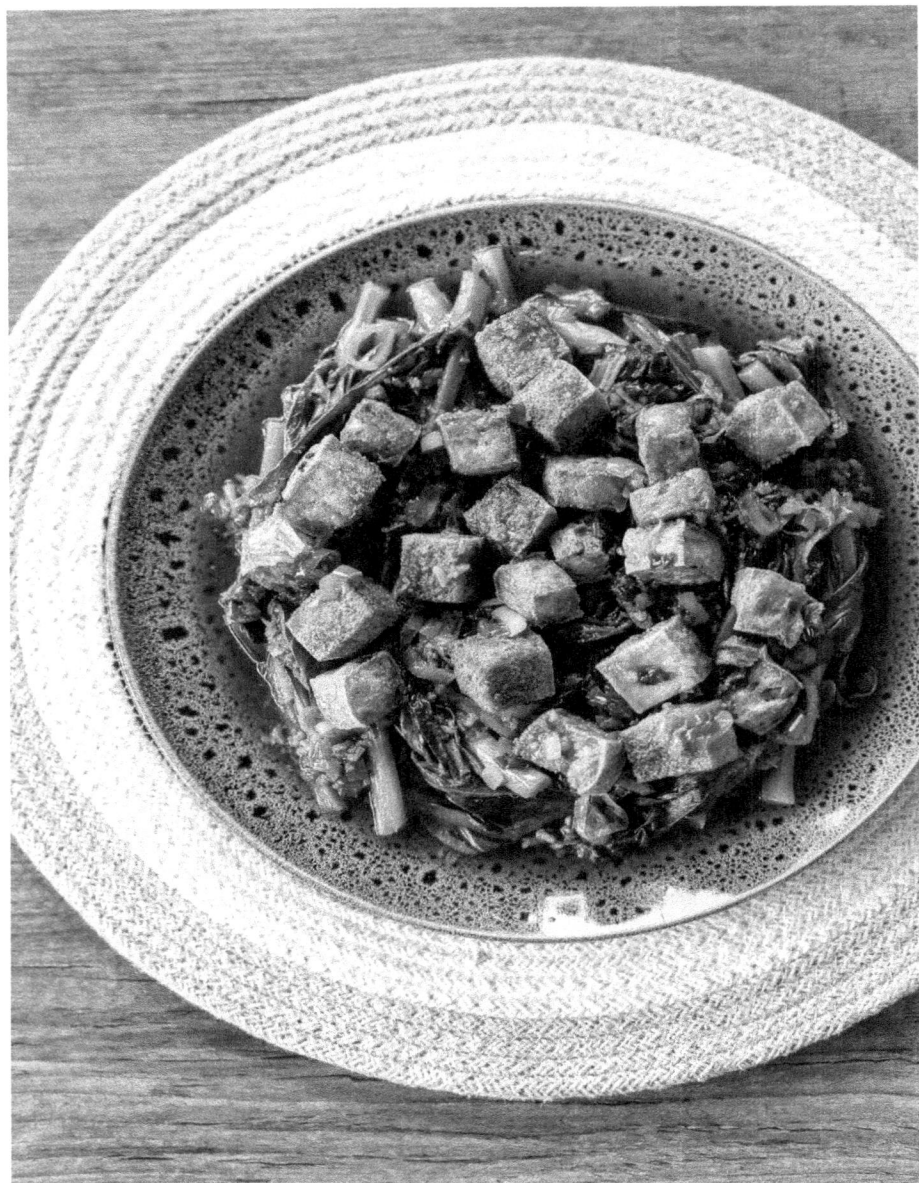

Air Fried Walnuts

Preparation Time:

10 minutes

Cooking Time:

5 minutes

Serve: 6

Ingredients:

2 cups walnuts
1 tsp olive oil
1/4 tsp garlic powder
1/4 tsp chili powder
Pepper Salt

Directions:

1.Add walnuts, garlic powder, chili powder, oil, pepper, and salt into the bowl and toss well.

2.Place the cooking tray in the air fryer basket. Line air fryer basket with parchment paper.

3.Select Air Fry mode. Set time to 5 minutes and temperature 320 F then press START.

4.The air fryer display will prompt you to ADD FOOD once the temperature is reached then place walnuts onto the parchment paper in the air fryer basket. Serve and enjoy.

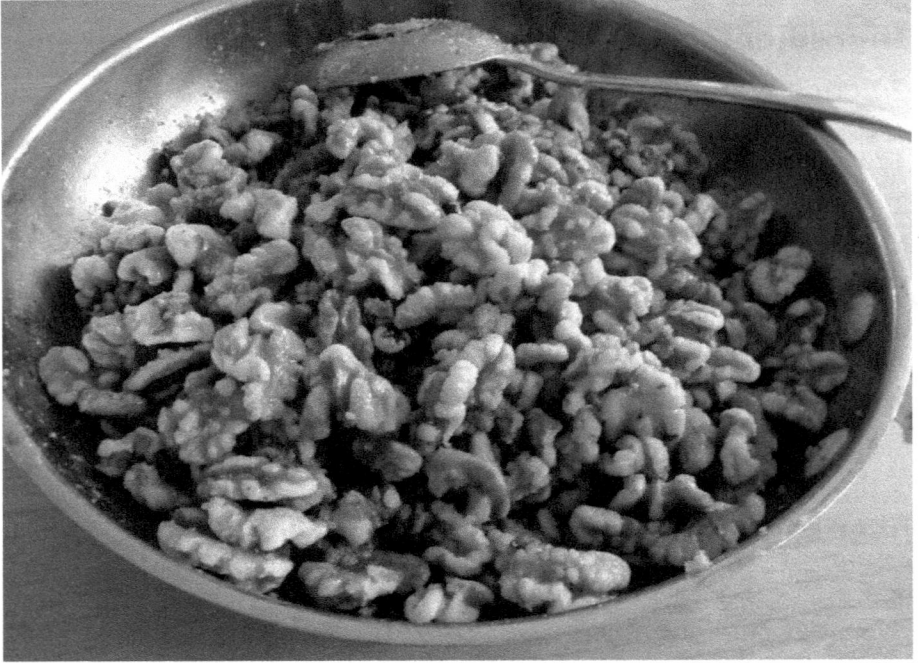

Parmesan Brussels Sprouts

Preparation Time:

10 minutes

Cooking Time:

12 minutes

Serve: 4

Ingredients:

1 lb Brussels sprouts, cut stems and halved
1 1/2 tbsp olive oil
1/4 cup parmesan cheese, grated
1/4 tsp garlic powder
1/4 tsp onion powder
Pepper Salt

Directions:

1.In a bowl, toss Brussels sprouts with oil, garlic powder, onion powder, pepper, and salt.

2.Place the cooking tray in the air fryer basket. Line air fryer basket with parchment paper. Select Air Fry mode.

3.Set time to 12 minutes and temperature 350 F then press START.

4.The air fryer display will prompt you to ADD FOOD once the temperature is reached then spread brussels sprouts onto the parchment paper in the air fryer basket. Top with grated parmesan cheese and serve.

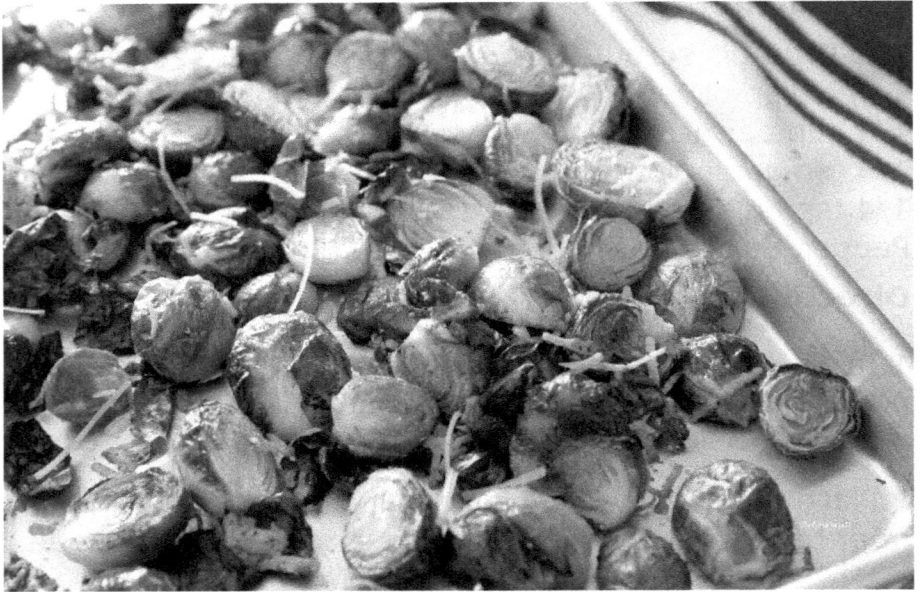

Stuffed Chicken Jalapenos

Preparation Time:

10 minutes

Cooking Time:

25 minutes

Serve: 12

Ingredients:

6 jalapenos, halved
1/2 cup chicken, cooked and shredded
1/4 tsp garlic powder
3 oz cream cheese
1/4 tsp dried oregano
1/4 cup green onion, sliced
1/4 cup Monterey jack cheese, shredded
1/4 tsp dried basil
1/4 tsp salt

Directions:

1.Mix all ingredients in a bowl except jalapenos.

2.Spoon 1 tablespoon mixture into each jalapeno half. Place the cooking tray in the air fryer basket.

3.Line air fryer basket with parchment paper. Select Bake mode. Set time to 25 minutes and temperature 390 F then press START.

4.The air fryer display will prompt you to ADD FOOD once the temperature is reached then place jalapeno halves onto the parchment paper in the air fryer basket. Serve and enjoy.

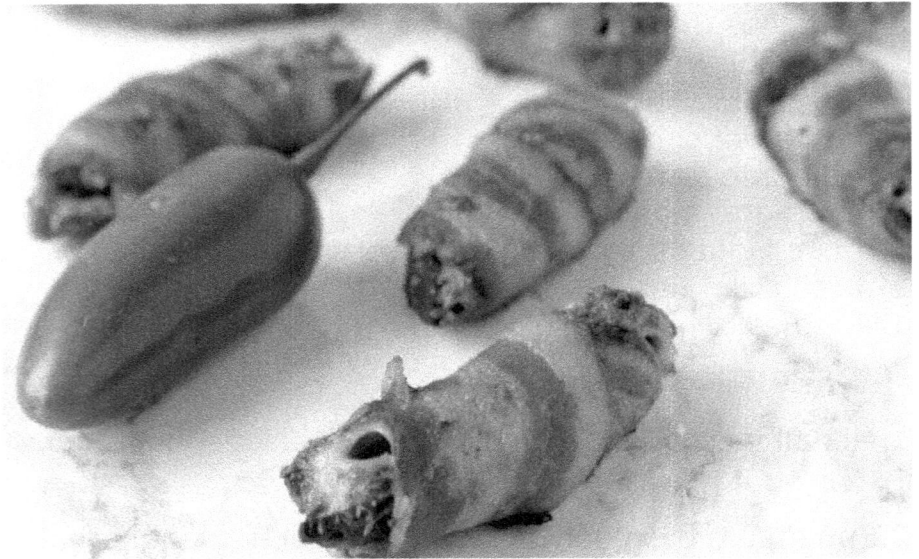

Spinach Sausage Balls

Preparation Time:

10 minutes

Cooking Time:

20 minutes

Serve: 10

Ingredients:

1egg
1/2 cup parmesan cheese, grated
1/2 cup mozzarella cheese, shredded
1 lb sausage
1 garlic clove, chopped
1/2 onion, chopped
1 cup spinach, chopped
1 tsp salt

Directions:

1.Add all ingredients in mixing bowl and mix until well combined.

2.Make balls from the mixture. Place the cooking tray in the air fryer basket.

3.Line air fryer basket with parchment paper. Select Bake mode. Set time to 20 minutes and temperature 400 F then press START.

4.The air fryer display will prompt you to ADD FOOD once the temperature is reached then place sausage balls onto the parchment paper in the air fryer basket. Serve and enjoy.

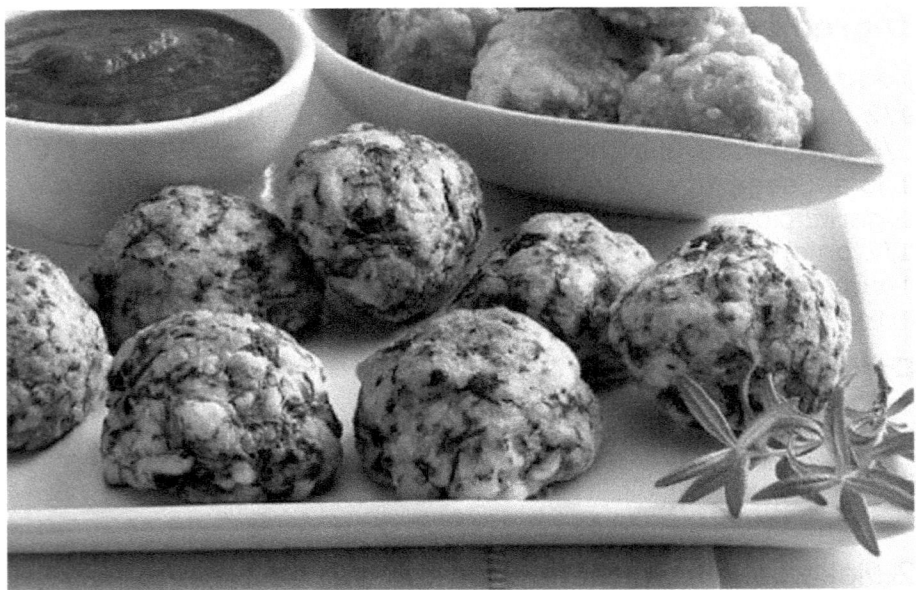

Crispy Zucchini Fries

Preparation Time:

10 minutes

Cooking Time:

20 minutes

Serve: 4

Ingredients:

1eggs
1 medium zucchini, peel and cut into matchsticks
1/4 tsp onion powder
1 cup pork rinds, crushed
1 tbsp heavy cream
1/2 cup parmesan cheese, grated
1/4 tsp garlic powder

Directions:

1.In a bowl, whisk together cream and eggs. In a shallow dish, mix together crushed pork rinds, parmesan cheese, onion powder, and garlic powder.

2.Dip each zucchini piece into the egg mixture then coat with pork rind mixture. Place the cooking tray in the air fryer basket.

3.Line air fryer basket with parchment paper. Select Bake mode. Set time to 20 minutes and temperature 400 F then press START.

4.The air fryer display will prompt you to ADD FOOD once the temperature is reached then place breaded zucchini fries onto the parchment paper in the air fryer basket. Serve and enjoy.

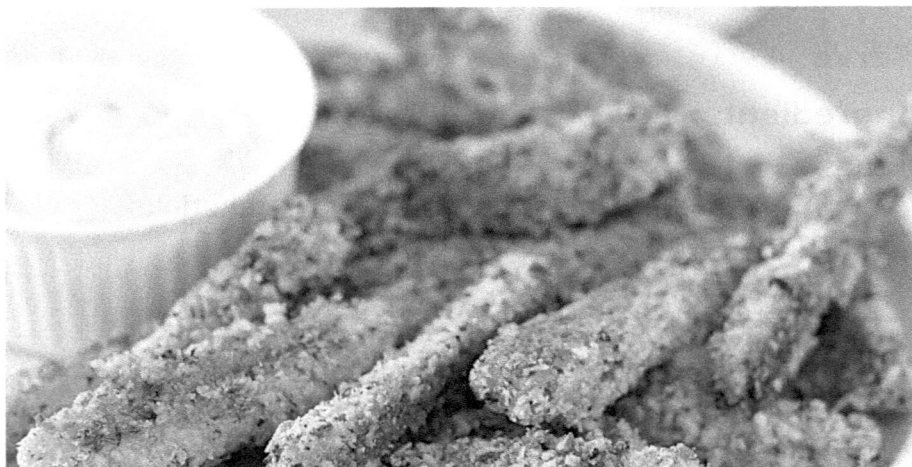

Cheesy Jalapeno Poppers

Preparation Time:

10 minutes

Cooking Time:

20 minutes

Serve: 24

Ingredients:

12 jalapeno peppers, cut in half and remove seeds
2 oz feta cheese
1/4 tsp garlic powder
1/2 tsp onion powder
1/4 cup cilantro, chopped
2 oz cheddar cheese, shredded
4 oz cream cheese

Directions:

1.Add all ingredients except jalapeno peppers into the bowl and mix well to combine.

2.Stuff cheese mixture into each jalapeno half. Place the cooking tray in the air fryer basket. Line air fryer basket with parchment paper.

3.Select Bake mode. Set time to 20 minutes and temperature 400 F then press START.

4.The air fryer display will prompt you to ADD FOOD once the temperature is reached then place jalapeno halves onto the parchment paper in the air fryer basket. Serve and enjoy

85

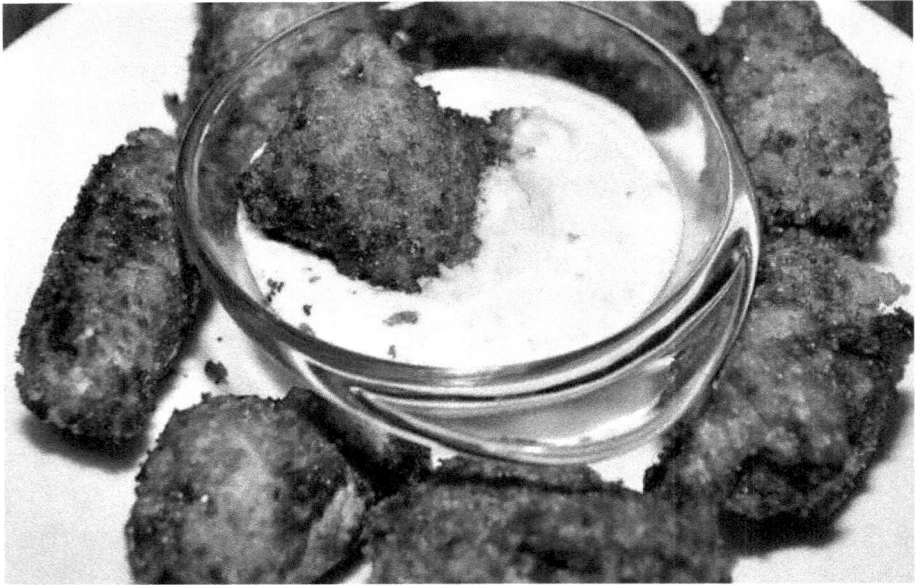

Roasted Cashew

Preparation Time:

5 minutes

Cooking Time:

10 minutes

Serve: 3

Ingredients:

3/4 cups cashews
1/2 tsp olive oil
1/2 tsp chili powder
1/4 tsp salt

Directions

1.Add all ingredients into the bowl and toss well. Place the cooking tray in the air fryer basket. Line air fryer basket with parchment paper. Select Bake mode.

2.Set time to 10 minutes and temperature 250 F then press START.

3.The air fryer display will prompt you to ADD FOOD once the temperature is reached then place cashews onto the parchment paper in the air fryer basket. Serve and enjoy.

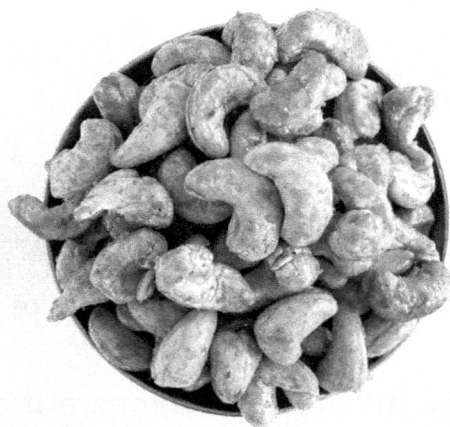

Lamb Patties

Preparation Time:

10 minutes

Cooking Time:

8 minutes

Serve: 4

Ingredients:

1lb ground lamb
1/4 cup fresh parsley, chopped
1tsp dried oregano
1cup feta cheese, crumbled
1tbsp garlic, minced
3basil leaves, minced
10 mint leaves, minced
1 jalapeno pepper, minced
1/4 tsp pepper
1/2 tsp kosher salt

Directions:

1.Add all ingredients into the mixing bowl and mix until well combined.

2.Make four equal shape patties from the meat mixture. Place the cooking tray in the air fryer basket. Line air fryer basket with parchment paper. Select Bake mode.

3.Set time to 8 minutes and temperature 390 F then press START.

4.The air fryer display will prompt you to ADD FOOD once the temperature is reached then place patties onto the parchment paper in the air fryer basket. Serve and enjoy

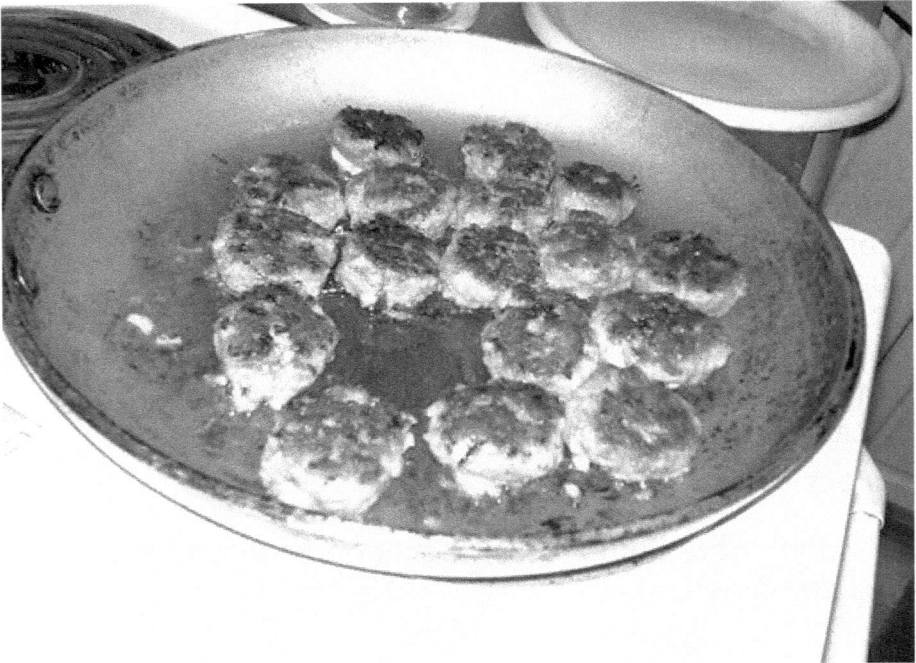

Buffalo Chicken Dip

Preparation Time:

10 minutes

Cooking Time:

25 minutes

Serve: 8

Ingredients:

1chicken breasts, skinless, boneless, cooked and shredded 1 cup Monterey jack cheese, shredded
1/2 cup ranch dressing
1/2 cup buffalo wing sauce
8oz cream cheese, softened
1 cup cheddar cheese, shredded
1/4 cup blue cheese, crumbled

Directions:

1.Add cream cheese into the baking dish and top with shredded chicken, ranch dressing, and buffalo sauce.

2.Sprinkle cheddar cheese, Monterey jack cheese, and blue cheese on top of chicken mixture. Cover dish with foil.

3.Select Bake mode. Set time to 25 minutes and temperature 350 F then press START.

4.The air fryer display will prompt you to ADD FOOD once the temperature is reached then place the baking dish in the air fryer basket. Serve and enjoy.

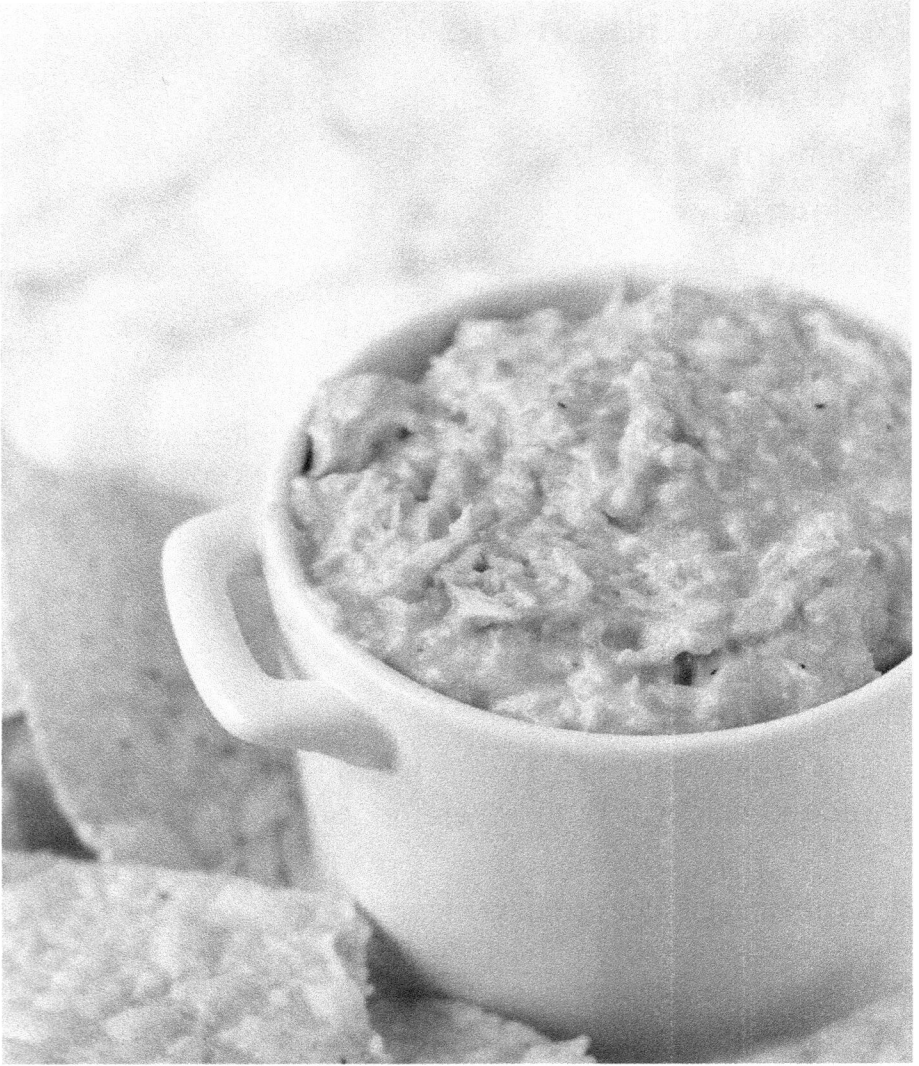

Ricotta Dip

Preparation Time:

10 minutes

Cooking Time:

15 minutes

Serve: 8

Ingredients:

1 cup ricotta cheese
1/2 tbsp fresh rosemary
1 tbsp lemon juice
2 tbsp olive oil
2 garlic cloves, minced
1/4 cup parmesan cheese
1/2 cup mozzarella cheese
Pepper Salt

Directions:

1.Add ricotta cheese, garlic, oil, lemon juice, rosemary, pepper, and salt into the baking dish and mix until well combined.

2.Sprinkle mozzarella cheese and parmesan cheese on top. Cover dish with foil. Select Bake mode.

3.Set time to 15 minutes and temperature 400 F then press START. The air fryer display will prompt you to ADD FOOD once the temperature is reached then place the baking dish in the air fryer basket. Serve and enjoy.

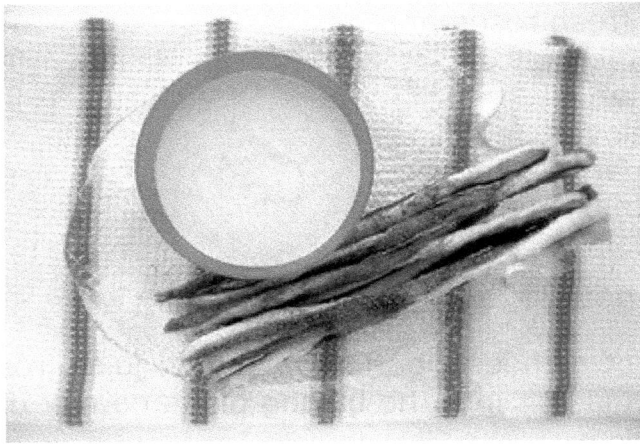

Spicy Artichoke Dip

Preparation Time:

10 minutes

Cooking Time:

30 minutes

Serve: 12

Ingredients:

1oz can green chiles, diced
15 oz can artichoke hearts, drained and chopped
2 cups mayonnaise
8 oz parmesan cheese, grated

Directions:

1.Add all ingredients into the mixing bowl and mix until well combined. Pour mixture into the 2-quart baking dish.

2.Cover dish with foil. Select Bake mode. Set time to 30 minutes and temperature 325 F then press START.

3.The air fryer display will prompt you to ADD FOOD once the temperature is reached then place the baking dish in the air fryer basket. Serve and enjoy.

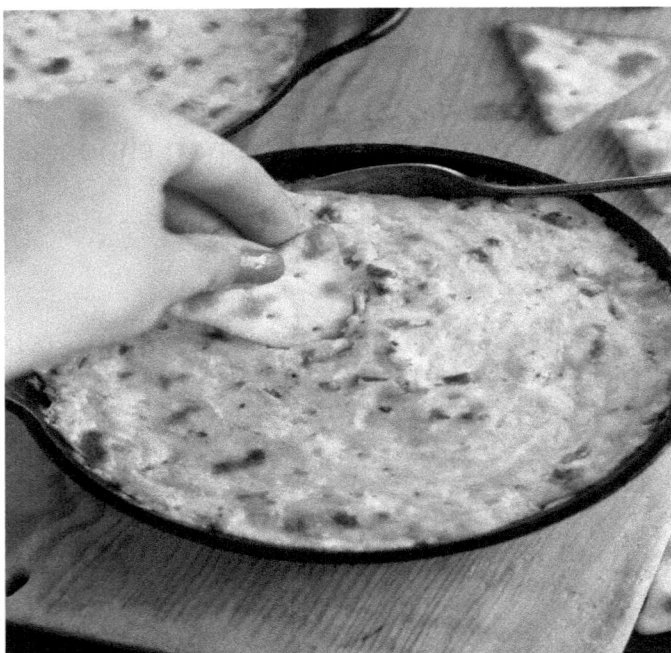

Fresh Herb Mushrooms

Preparation Time:

10 minutes

Cooking Time:

14 minutes

Serve: 4

Ingredients:

1 lb mushrooms
1 tbsp basil, minced
1 garlic clove, minced
1/2 tbsp vinegar
1/2 tsp ground coriander
1 tsp rosemary, chopped
Pepper Salt

Directions:

1.Add all ingredients into the large bowl and toss well.

2.Place the cooking tray in the air fryer basket. Line air fryer basket with parchment paper. Select Bake mode.

3.Set time to 14 minutes and temperature 350 F then press START.

4.The air fryer display will prompt you to ADD FOOD once the temperature is reached then spread mushrooms onto the parchment paper in the air fryer basket. Serve and enjoy.

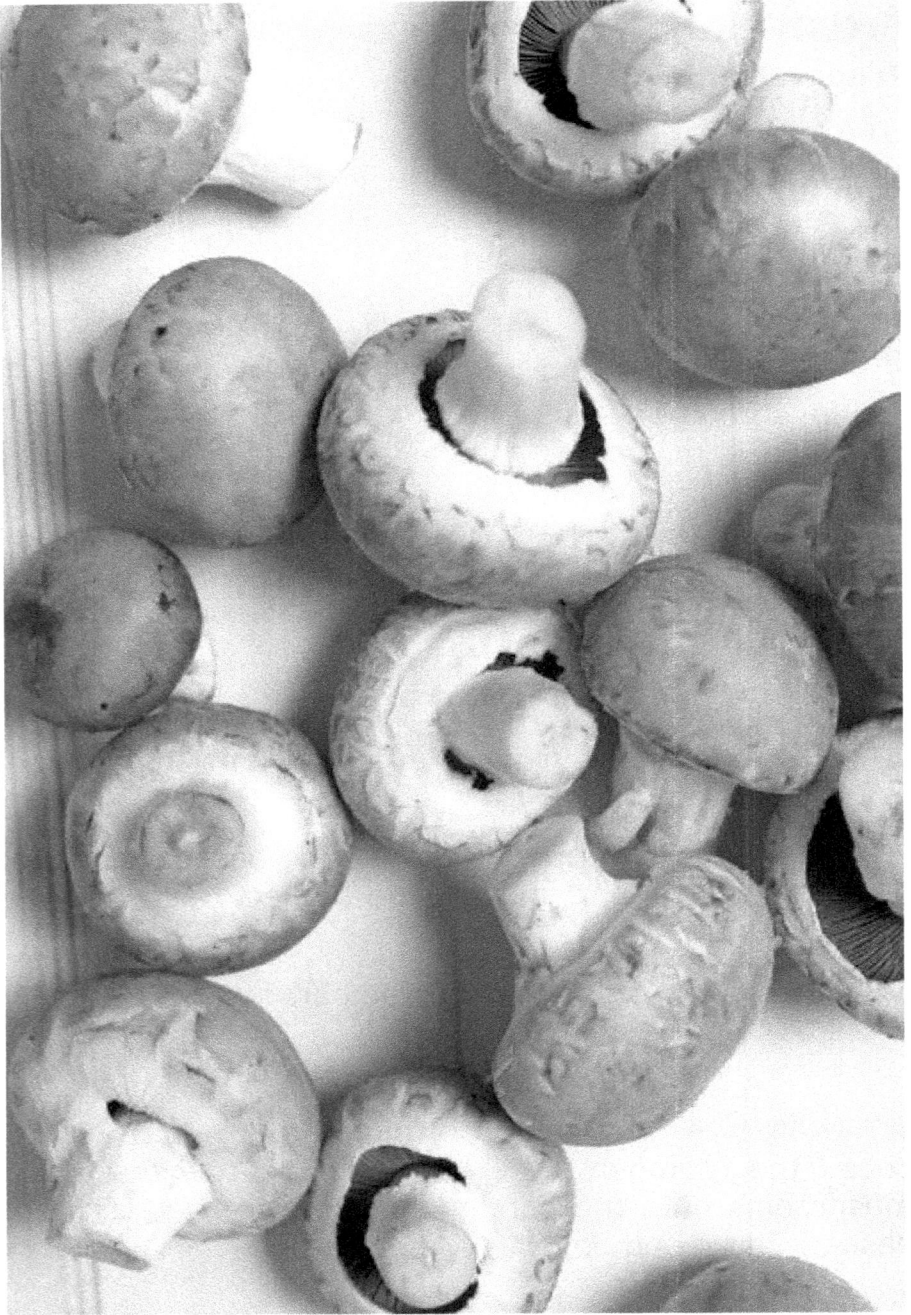

Zucchini Dill Dip

Preparation Time:

10 minutes

Cooking Time:

15 minutes

Serve: 6

Ingredients:

1 lb zucchini, grated & squeeze out all liquid

1 tsp garlic, minced

1 tsp dill, chopped

1 tbsp lime juice

1 tbsp olive oil

1 cup heavy cream

Pepper Salt

Directions:

1.Add all ingredients into the large bowl and mix until well combined.

2.Pour zucchini mixture into the prepared baking dish. Select Bake mode. Set time to 15 minutes and temperature 375 F then press START.

3.The air fryer display will prompt you to ADD FOOD once the temperature is reached then place the baking dish in the air fryer basket. Serve and enjoy.

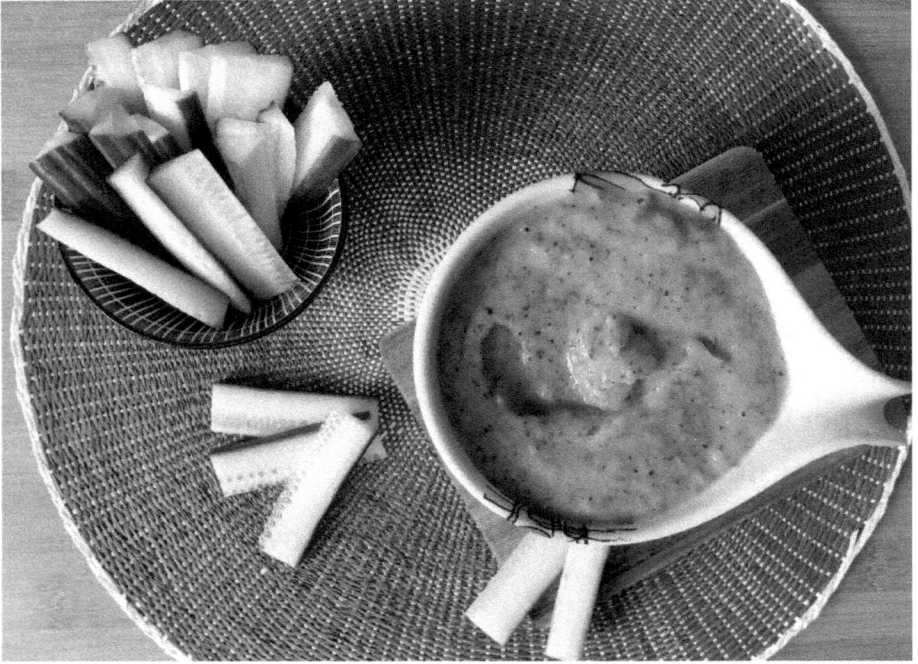

Cheddar Cheese Garlic Dip

Preparation Time:

10minutes

Cooking Time:

8 minutes

Serve: 6

Ingredients:

13 oz cheddar cheese, remove the rind and cubed
4   garlic cloves, chopped
1 tbsp dried thyme
2 tsp rosemary, chopped
Pepper Salt

Directions:

1.Add all ingredients into the mixing bowl and mix well.

2.Pour mixture into the baking dish and cover dish with foil.

3.Select Bake mode. Set time to 8 minutes and temperature 375 F then press START.

4.The air fryer display will prompt you to ADD FOOD once the temperature is reached then place the baking dish in the air fryer basket. Serve and enjoy.

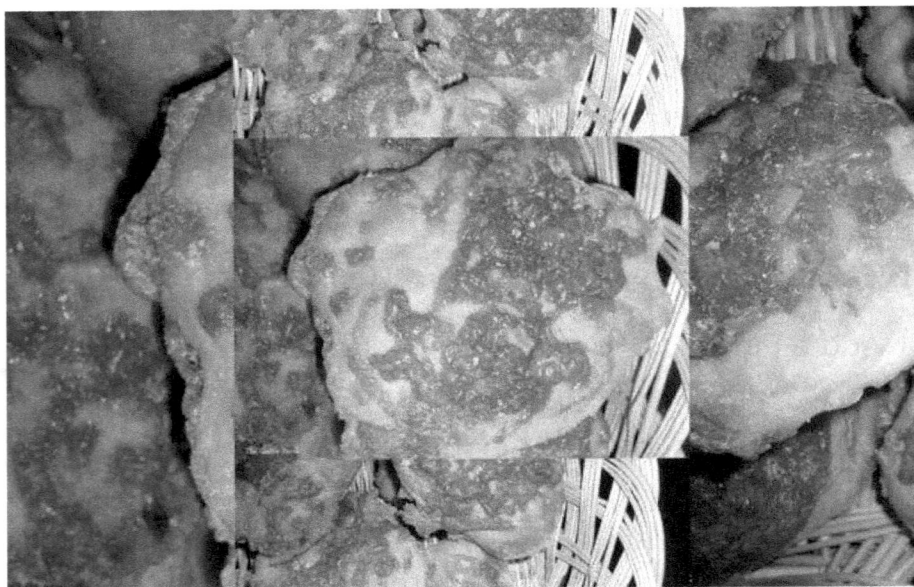

Air Fry Taro Fries

Preparation Time:

10 minutes

Cooking Time:

20 minutes

Serve: 2

Ingredients:

7small taro, peel and cut into fries shape
1 tbsp olive oil
1/2 tsp chili powder
1/4 tsp garlic powder
1/4 tsp pepper
1/2 tsp salt

Directions:

1.Add taro fries in a bowl and drizzle with olive oil. Season with chili powder, garlic powder, pepper, and salt.

2.Place the cooking tray in the air fryer basket. Line air fryer basket with parchment paper. Select Bake mode.

3.Set time to 20 minutes and temperature 375 F then press START.

4.The air fryer display will prompt you to ADD FOOD once the temperature is reached then place taro fries onto the parchment paper in the air fryer basket. Serve and enjoy.

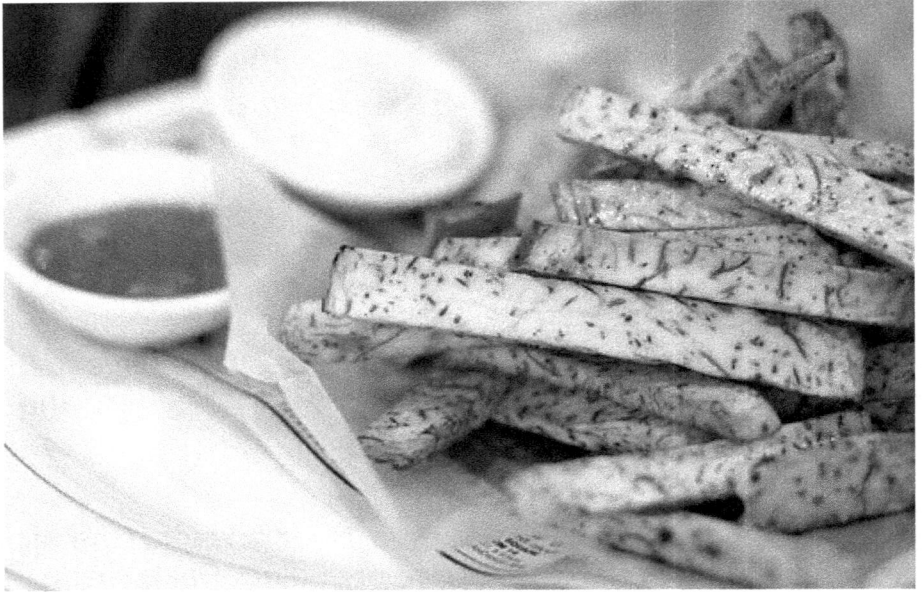

Crispy Zucchini Chips

Preparation Time:

10 minutes

Cooking Time:

30 minutes

Serve: 2

Ingredients:

2 medium zucchini, cut into
1/4-inch thick slices
1/2 cup parmesan cheese, grated
1/4 cup olive oil
Pepper Salt

Directions:

1.In a mixing bowl, toss zucchini slices with cheese, oil, pepper, and salt. Place the cooking tray in the air fryer basket.

2.Line air fryer basket with parchment paper. Select Bake mode.

Set time to 30 minutes and temperature 300 F then press START.

3.The air fryer display will prompt you to ADD FOOD once the temperature is reached then arrange zucchini slices onto the parchment paper in the air fryer basket.

4.Turn halfway through. Serve and enjoy.

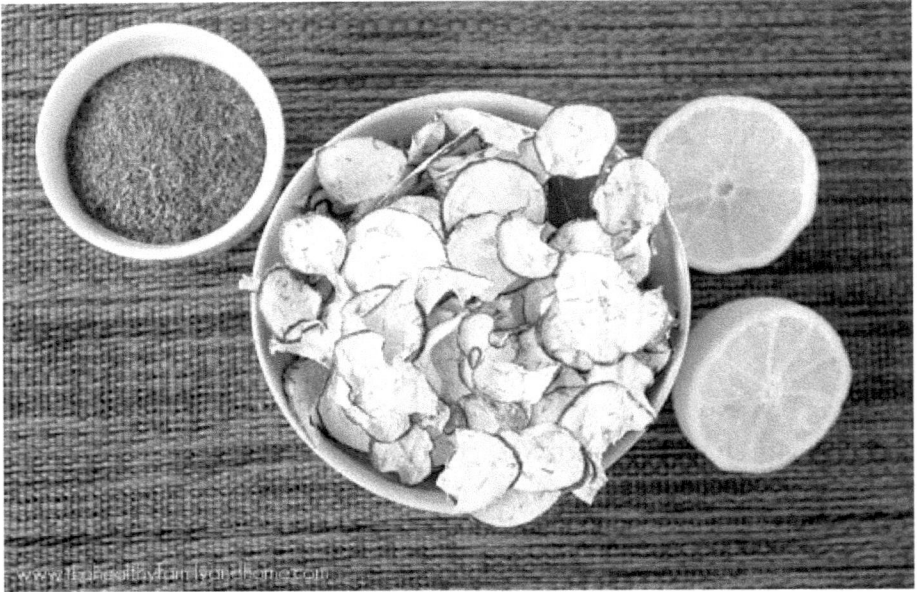

Cinnamon Apple Chips

Preparation Time:

10 minutes

Cooking Time:

8minutes

Serve: 4

Ingredients:

1 large apple, sliced thinly
1/4 tsp ground nutmeg
1/4 tsp ground cinnamon

Directions:

1.Season apple slices with nutmeg and cinnamon. Place the cooking tray in the air fryer basket. Line air fryer basket with parchment paper.

2.Select Air Fry mode. Set time to 8 minutes and temperature 375 F then press START.

3.The air fryer display will prompt you to ADD FOOD once the temperature is reached then place apple slices onto the parchment paper in the air fryer basket. Serve and enjoy.

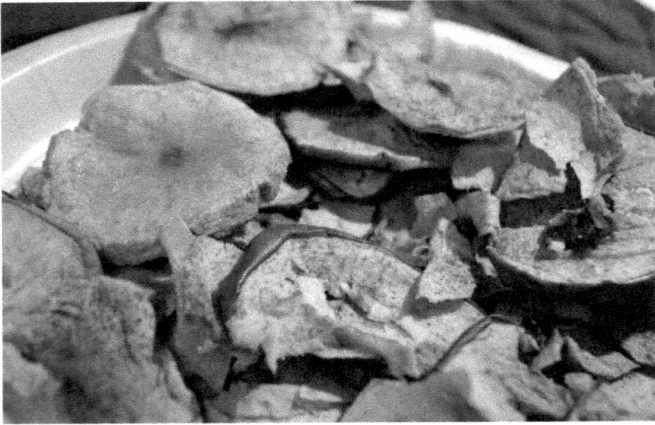

Easy Sausage Balls

Preparation Time:

10 minutes

Cooking Time:

16 minutes

Serve: 10

Ingredients:

1cup almond flour
1 lb ground sausage
1 cup cheddar cheese, shredded

Directions:

1.Add all ingredients into the mixing bowl and mix until well combined.

2.Make 1-inch balls from meat mixture. Place the cooking tray in the air fryer basket. Place piece of aluminum foil into the air fryer basket.

3.Select Air Fry mode. Set time to 16 minutes and temperature 375 F then press START.

4.The air fryer display will prompt you to ADD FOOD once the temperature is reached then place meatballs onto the aluminum foil in the air fryer basket. Serve and enjoy.

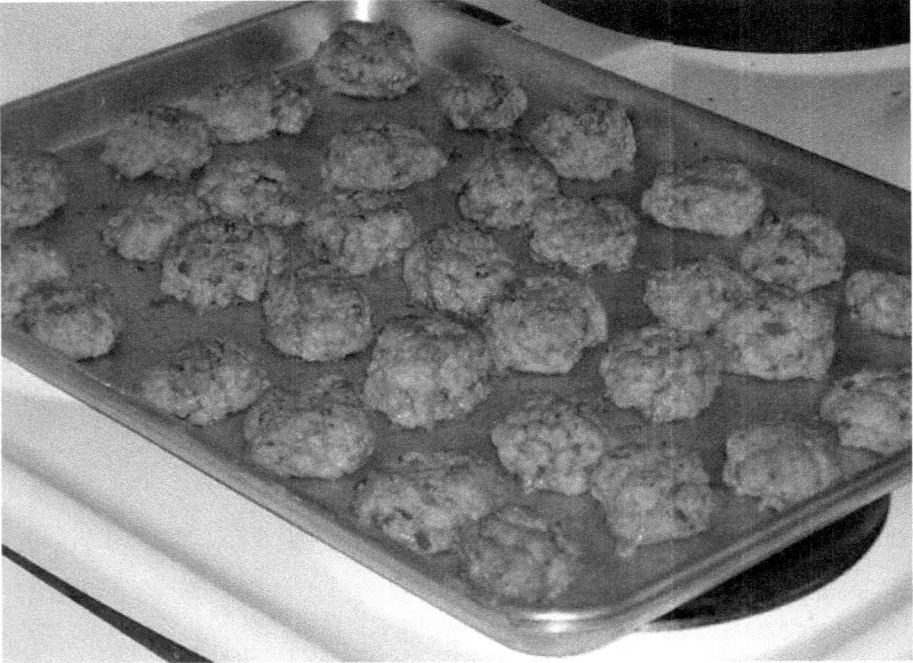

www.ingramcontent.com/pod-product-compliance
Lightning Source LLC
Chambersburg PA
CBHW070723030426

42336CB00013B/1907